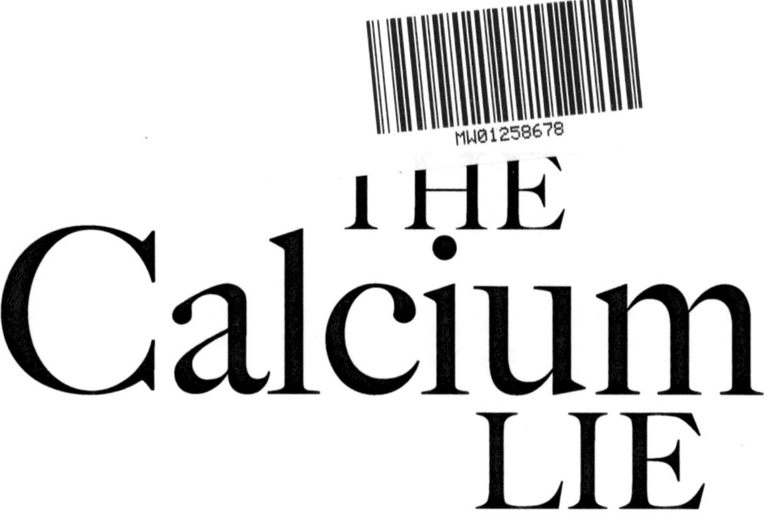

THE Calcium LIE

WHAT YOUR DOCTOR DOESN'T KNOW COULD **KILL** YOU

ROBERT THOMPSON, M.D. • KATHLEEN BARNES

INTRUTHPRESS
Brevard, North Carolina

The purpose of this book is to educate. It is not intended to serve as a replacement for professional medical advice. Any use of this information in this book is at the reader's discretion. This book is sold with the understanding that neither the publisher nor the authors have any liability or responsibility for any injury caused or alleged to be caused directly or indirectly by the information contained in this book. While every effort has been made to ensure its accuracy, the book's contents should not be construed as medical advice. To obtain medical advice on your individual health needs, please consult a qualified health care practitioner.

Published by InTruth Press

www.intruthpress.com • e-mail: InTruthPress@citcom.net

Library of Congress Cataloging-in-Publication Data

Thompson, Robert
Barnes, Kathleen
The Calcium Lie: What Your Doctor Doesn't Know Could Kill You
p. cm.
Includes bibliographic references and index.
ISBN 978-0-981581859
Library of Congress Control Number: 2008927243

Graphic design: Gary A. Rosenberg
Cover design: Brion Sausser, Book Creatives

Manufactured in the United States of America.

Contents

Dedications

To my precious family, immediate and extended, I love you all. Without your continued support and love, life becomes more difficult. There are many ways to count our blessings. You bring much joy and immeasurable wealth to each and every day of my life.

To my children, Nathan and Tiffany, it has been a privilege beyond compare to watch you grow, and to see you blossom. I am proud to know you let alone to call you my children. Thank you for your love, your courage, and for making great choices and living lives of distinction, character, and integrity. You make a Dad smile.

To my patients and mentors for teaching me and challenging me, and to my Lord for the wisdom, blessings, and salvation you have given me, I am eternally grateful and thankful. May this book bring honor and glory to your name through my life.

—Dr. Robert Thompson

For Joe, as always, with all my heart.

—Kathleen Barnes

Foreword

DR. ROBERT THOMPSON IS AN ENLIGHTENED PHYSICIAN.

His medical education gave him the knowledge of human physiology and biochemistry that he needed to become a competent physician. Dr. Thompson is among the elite, however, because his education did not end after graduation, but has continued throughout his career.

He became enlightened when he used his medical and scientific knowledge to surpass the knowledge of most other doctors, and formulated nutritional concepts based on basic scientific truths that are effective in treating and, dare I say, curing diseases that conventional medicine proclaims incurable.

Dr. Thompson is enlightened because of his unending dedication to helping his patients return to health and his passion for finding answers to his patients' health challenges.

Robert Thompson is a doctor in the true sense of the word. He is a teacher, as evidenced by his writings. Beyond all else, *The Calcium Lie* is intended to teach. Not only does this remarkable book teach about the intricate workings of the human body, it is also thought provoking.

The Calcium Lie can aid the average individual to understand and make sense of the complexities of the body in a down-to-earth fashion. This knowledge helps us to begin to ask questions about our health care rather than just accepting the status quo.

The Calcium Lie is a call to action to everyone who wants to become involved in and take responsibility for his own health.

Dr. Thompson's enlightenment is also demonstrated in the pioneering spirit of this book. The information contained herein is the wave of the future, because it teaches that we are individuals, and that therapeutic intervention should be based upon the individual need, and not merely a condition or disease process.

Dr. Thompson's viewpoint is certain to be controversial. It is my sincere hope that all readers, patients and physicians alike, carefully review the information offered here and recognize its value.

—David L. Watts, D.C. Ph.D., F.A.C.E.P.
CEO of Trace Elements, Inc., Addison, Texas

Preface

I AM A CARING DOCTOR WHO WENT to medical school with altruistic ideas and a belief in doing the right thing. When I completed my medical training, I greeted my chosen career with great excitement about practicing medicine on the cutting edge and doing the best job I could do for my patients.

Over the next few years, I grew increasingly disenchanted with my profession and with the uncharitable attitudes of many of my colleagues, who frequently resisted basic science and medical advances in the name of protecting their status quo. Even a local hospital where I worked was unhappy with me when some of my more advanced procedures resulted in outpatient, rather than inpatient, surgeries and shortened hospital stays. It really burst my idealistic new doctor bubble to learn that this hospital wanted its patients to stay in longer no matter what the trauma to the patient, because—"ca-ching"—the hospitals make more money that way. Today, of course, outpatient surgery has become commonplace.

Finally, in 1996, I decided I was going to quit medicine. I was looking around for another career when I was notified I had been chosen to be listed in an exclusive peer-reviewed directory, "Best Doctors in America".

I was overwhelmed by the honor, and the irony, that the honor came at a time when I had decided to hang up my stethoscope for good. Maybe all that training was not a waste after all. I took it as a sign that I was to remain in the medical profession.

I took it as a call back to my medical school training and ideals, and to some of the basic scientific concepts I seemed to have lost in the intervening years. That was an epiphany for me, and an opportunity for me to take a new look at the way I was treating my patients.

I first realized that many of my pregnant patients were taking supplements and that, in order to be conscientious about their treatment, I needed to know more about them: what was good, what was bad, what worked, what didn't and how much to take. I began to do my own research to find out which ones were safe and which ones weren't.

That opened the door for me. I began learning about herbs and homeopathics and other natural treatments. I continued to grow and evolve in this process over the next few years, helping patients in new ways, often getting the same results with herbs and homeopathics as with prescription drugs, but with less toxicity and fewer side effects.

I soon realized that I was still treating my patients' symptoms, perhaps with less toxicity, but nevertheless, like most doctors, I wasn't treating the underlying causes of their symptoms. I began to be more aware of the impact of nutrition in this equation. That opened new insights for me about the supplements people were taking, what was true about human nutrition and, more importantly, what was not true. Eventually, I discovered The Calcium Lie, The Vitamin Lie and The Mineral Lies and began to realize their impact on my patients' health and disease processes.

Along the way, I discovered what worked and what helped people get better and what didn't. As I continued to make recommendations to patients, I saw them continually getting better and overcoming their health problems. This is what we physicians were supposed to be doing all along, what a concept!

I was especially pleased to find ways to help my patients with Type 2 diabetes and insulin resistance to overcome their blood sugar problems on a long-term basis. Were they "cured" of their diabetes? Maybe not, but what else can you call it when they have no symptoms and their laboratory tests and blood sugars remain in the normal range over many years?

I was tremendously excited about my discoveries. Unfortunately, I didn't find other caring physicians who shared my passion and were willing to listen to my ideas. Then I began attending meetings of the American College for Advancement in Medicine (ACAM), and another new world opened for me. In ACAM, I found like-minded doctors who realized there were better ways to treat patients and who were motivated to find and share them.

I'm not a zealot. I believe there are many good elements to conventional medicine. There are good medications, fantastic surgeries and cures, and amazing advancements that were not available a decade or two ago. We don't need to throw out the baby with the bathwater.

However, our current medical system is not only exorbitantly expensive, it has created a system in which doctors are reimbursed for allowing people to get sick rather than for keeping them healthy.

There is something elementally wrong with a system in which an insurance company will pay to amputate the leg of a diabetic patient rather than address the healing with nutritional therapies—at less cost. This is a travesty of everything we stand for as physicians, as Americans and as caring people.

Unfortunately, the nutrition industry also has its flaws. Its focus is largely about sales. It is quite similar to the pharmaceutical industry in many respects, but once again, there are some amazing supplements on the market today. They can produce good results for you if you take the right ones. There is also tremendous waste here. Exorbitant amounts of money are spent on supplements that have little or no nutritional value or health benefit. I realized that, just as I would try to pick out the best medication for treating a medical problem, I needed to be accountable for trying to help my patients pick out the best supplements to make up for the tremendous deficiencies in our food. Most patients would prefer to get better instead of having me treat their symptoms.

In the end, patients and physicians are going to have to realize that withholding of care and rationing of care are likely to become commonplace because, as a society, we simply cannot afford to pay for all the health crises we are developing as our population ages.

For the past six years, colleagues have urged me to write this book. So here, it is—finally! I'm putting this information out there for patients and physicians alike to learn from it and grow into greater health. There are many books out there, however, we believe this one is unique.

The exposure of The Calcium Lie is huge in terms of its potential impact on health care, now and in the future. It's a change in medical practice recommendations that can't take place fast enough.

To the best of our ability, we have made an attempt to provide truth, facts and reliable information, in simple terms and in ways the average person can understand.

My co-author, Kathleen Barnes, and I have written this book together, although much of it is in first person based on my experience.

Kathleen Barnes is a health journalist with great depth of experience, not only in conventional medical research and terminology, but through the passion she has had for natural health for more than 30 years. She is author or editor of 13 books, most of them on natural health subjects, and she wrote a weekly natural health column for Woman's World magazine for more than six years. Her ability to help translate complex medical terminology into simple and easily understandable terms has helped me to stay on the "straight and narrow" when I threatened to get too technical in my concepts.

If you've read this book and it resonates with you, tell a friend. Give a copy to a friend. Copy the last chapter and give it to your doctor, with our blessing. Better yet, buy a copy as a gift for your doctor. You, and your fellow patients, will reap the benefits.

We wish you all the best in your quest to regain your health. If you use the principles in this book, we have no doubt you will succeed.

—Robert Thompson, M.D.

Introduction

WE ARE ALL VICTIMS OF HEALTH LIES. These lies, held with an almost religious zealotry, are quite literally killing us.

Primary among those lies is the notion that bones are made of calcium, with the dogmatic exhortation from almost every doctor on the planet that we all need supplemental calcium in order to have strong bones. This is absolutely untrue and without any reliable scientific evidence. In fact, our bones are made of at least 12 minerals, including calcium, and we need all of them in proper proportions in order to have healthy bones and a healthy metabolism.

From this scientifically unfounded supposition comes a cascade of health consequences that are nothing less than devastating.

We've written this book from a place of passionate conviction that our collective health is at risk from The Calcium Lie and a handful of other lies to which we are all subjected.

We hope the truths in this book will lead you to a new life of exceptional health.

—Robert Thompson, M.D., Soldotna, Alaska

—Kathleen Barnes, Brevard, North Carolina

CHAPTER 1

Minerally Bankrupt

THERE'S A BIG LIE THAT HAS SUCKED US ALL IN, consumers and medical professionals alike. That Big Lie is killing us.

What's the lie?

It started with a wild notion that calcium is essential for strong bones. Nearly all of us and our doctors have bought into this "Calcium Lie," hook line and sinker. We believe that unless we get loads of calcium, our bones will crumble to powder. It's not true. It's never been true and basic science taught in every university in the world shows us the error of this belief system.

Before we go any further, let us tell you that calcium is only one of at least 12 minerals that build strong bones.

If you take calcium to strengthen your bones, you are signing your own death warrant. Think of this: Calcium hardens concrete. Imagine what it can harden in your body!

What caused us to buy into The Calcium Lie and how are we paying for the error of our ways? Here's the story:

The invention of the refrigerator was the beginning of humankind's modern health crisis.

In 1876, the first practical refrigerator was invented and refrigerators became commonly available by the turn of the century.

So why did this cause a health crisis for humankind?

The answer is simple: We stopped using sea salt to preserve meat and other foods and thereby robbed our bodies of the essential minerals we need to survive and thrive. No matter that medical science has flourished in the past century with advances ranging from the invention of synthetic insulin to antibiotics to CAT scans, MRIs, robotic surgery and more.

These medical miracles may all have their places, but without the basic building blocks of nutrition that we need to maintain, sustain and repair our bodies, we humans are never going to find the vibrant health that is our birthright.

At the moment, this is a squandered birthright. However, we can begin to regain our health by simple and affordable means. In the process, we can treat and eliminate some of the greatest health challenges of our time: obesity, diabetes, atherosclerosis (hardening of the arteries), hypertension, hypothyroidism, osteoporosis, depression, migraines and more.

How? The answer is so simple it will surprise you.

All we have to do is add minerals as natural salts to our diets in the forms of sea salt and rock salt, as food and in supplemental form.

PAINLESS BIOCHEMISTRY

Please bear with us for a few paragraphs while we review with you the basic science that underlies this astonishing shortsightedness on the part of humankind, and specifically on the part of the medical profession. We have all failed to understand and recognize the importance of basic biochemistry that lies at the heart of the medical conditions that plague modern humans.

You probably already know that our bodies are mainly water. On the average, 72% of your body weight is water, pure and simple. If you weigh 150 pounds, you have 108 pounds of water in your body. This is a basic premise of our physiology: Anything we put in our bodies MUST be water soluble or have a specific transport mechanism to be absorbed.

The remainder of your body weight is minerals. All 28% of it. For a 150-pound person, this means we're carrying around 42 pounds of a life-giving soup of 78 minerals, ranging from the commonly known calcium, magnesium, sodium and potassium to the more esoteric chromium, manganese, selenium and copper, to the more rare trace minerals like fluorine, cobalt, germanium and molybdenum, to name a few.

Bear with us. This is getting exciting.

Now, the planet's oceans and salt beds contain all of the minerals and trace minerals we need to be in perfect health.

Sea salt and rock salt contain all of the minerals in the exact proportion that our bodies require (except sodium, more about that later). Quite simply, these minerals are necessary for every single body function to work: biochemical, electrical, chemical and physiological.

We don't know about you, but we find this awe inspiring, miraculous and perhaps one of the strongest scientific arguments for the existence of an intelligent creative force that is beyond our comprehension.

WE'RE GOING DOWNHILL

Getting back to the refrigerator, when we stopped preserving our food with naturally occurring salts, we became progressively deficient in some, if not all, of those essential minerals. Because a chemical "fingerprint" is passed from mother to child (more about that in Chapter 6), each generation has become progressively more deficient in these essential minerals.

At about the same time, humankind in all of its wisdom began to severely deplete the soil in which we grow our food. The introduction of chemical fertilizers actually robbed and depleted the soil of its nutrients.

In the same general time frame, we wise humans began to build huge dams to control and reduce natural flooding. We might think that was a good idea, but it wasn't, since floodwaters actually carry essential mineral nutrients back into the land. Plants grown in these minerally poor soils were increasingly unable to extract the nutrients into their fruits and bring them to our tables.

In 1936, the U.S. Senate actually warned the population that our soil was seriously depleted of minerals. The warning was based on research from such prestigious academic institutions as Yale, Rutgers, Johns Hopkins and Columbia, in conjunction with the U.S. Department of Agriculture.

Dr. Charles Northern, one of the lead researchers in these projects, issued a prophetic warning at the time: ". . . Countless human ills stem from the fact that impoverished soil of America no longer provides plant foods with mineral elements essential to human nourishment and health. Millions of acres no longer contain the valuable trace elements . . . It is not commonly realized, however, that vitamins control the body's appropriation of minerals, and in the absence of minerals they have no function to perform. Lacking vitamins, the system can make some use of minerals, but lacking minerals, vitamins are useless."

Decades later, Dr. Northern's warning was underscored by Dr. Linus

Pauling, winner of two Nobel prizes, who said, "You can trace every sickness, every disease and every ailment to a mineral deficiency."

Clearly the warnings fell on deaf ears.

Since then, the problem has gotten worse. A 1992 Earth Summit report placed the decline in mineral content of North American soils at 85% and seven years later, in 1999, a Rutgers University Study revealed the mineral content of commercial fruits and vegetables was less than 16% compared to vine ripened organic produce. Since the mineral content determines the vitamin content, our commercial produce has almost no nutritional value!

It's no wonder that we are sick when we take into account the fact that much of our produce has often been shipped thousands of miles, picked before prime ripeness and loses nutrients during shipping.

We'll go into the benefits of vine ripened and organic foods in coming chapters, but it's important to know now that the mineral content of vine ripened fruits and vegetables is substantially higher than that of commercially produced foods. So get vine ripened, fresh, raw, unheated, fresh frozen or dried fruits and vegetables, and go organic as much as you can! In winter, you can get some of your needs from raw nuts and seeds, but it will almost certainly be necessary for you to take a trace mineral supplement.

TABLE SALT IS A HEALTH DESTROYER

Then came the final blow: Early in the 20th century, more "scientific" advances brought us pretty white convenient table salt that was composed only of two minerals: sodium and chloride or sodium chloride. It was a fine and granular salt. It was convenient. Scientists of the time apparently considered the other 76 minerals present in rock salt and sea salt to be unnecessary and unsightly, so they were "purified" out.

The result: The first evidence of our grave error came in 1924 when we began to see iodine deficiency within our population, leading to the widespread development of thyroid goiter (enlargement of the thyroid gland and thyroid hormone deficiency). This led to the addition of another mineral, iodide or iodine, and our pretty white table salt became "iodized salt." It should have been our first clue that many other vital nutrients were missing when we began to refine our salt. But we failed to recognize the signals. Our collective downhill slide into widespread mineral deficiency began to accelerate.

Our bodies began to desperately seek the minerals we need to survive, to

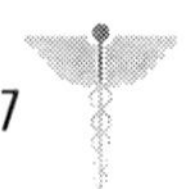

the point where they even drew on similar-acting minerals to try to duplicate the missing nutrients.

THE CALCIUM LIE IN BRIEF

The Mineral Lie was the first of many lies. *The Calcium Lie*, which is an outgrowth of the Mineral Lie, has led us to a host of health problems of untold proportions. We'll go into them in greater detail in the coming chapters, but here is the foundation of The Calcium Lie:

Most people, even many medical professionals, began to believe that bones are made of calcium. As we've said before, our bones are actually composed of at least 12 minerals. One of them is calcium, but a proper balance of all these minerals is essential for bone health, strong bones and the prevention of osteoporosis. By the way, osteoporosis is defined as a loss of minerals from the bones, not just calcium deficiency. Remember, calcium hardens concrete, not bones!

Our doctors told us we needed more calcium to keep our bones strong, so we started popping calcium supplements, adding calcium to many of our foods and we were told to drink at least two glasses of calcium-rich milk every day.

This gross oversimplification for the benefit of the dairy industry is similar to The Mineral Lie and the iodine story. What we've sacrificed in the name of simplification and convenience has led us to serious errors and the propagation of outright lies in an approach to health that has taken a devastating toll.

Ask yourself, what are your bones made of? What builds strong bones? What is osteoporosis, a loss of what from the bones? Almost everyone including educated medical personnel, dieticians, and even physicians, will all answer, "Calcium." That's The Calcium Lie.

This is a big mistake! We are so programmed to believe that bones are made of calcium it has almost become dogmatic.

Here's the truth: If you take calcium supplements and eat calcium-rich foods, (probably on the recommendation of your doctor), you'll build up excess calcium in your system coupled with mineral deficiencies and imbalances that will cause plaque in arteries, kidney stones, gallstones, bone spurs, osteoarthritis, hypertension, thyroid hormone resistance known as Type 2 hypothyroidism, obesity, Type 2 diabetes and many other diseases we'll address in this book.

When we took the sea salt and rock salt out of our diets, we lost about 15% of the nutritional value of our foods. Adding calcium to our diets to try to correct multiple mineral deficiencies and prevent or treat osteoporosis won't help. It will actually make your mineral imbalances worse. Excess calcium causes more deficiencies and imbalances. It doesn't correct fracture risks from osteoporosis. And it leads to a myriad of other nutritional problems and diseases.

Our belief that calcium is the essential element for strong bones is an erroneous idea that has turned into an outright lie. Today nearly all of us believe we need extra calcium to have healthy bones and to prevent osteoporosis. More is better, so we add calcium. It is added to everything from orange juice to cereal, sports drinks to baby food, soy-based drinks and pasta. The list is endless. We need minerals. We need all of them, not just one mineral.

Worst of all, we feed our children calcium-rich milk in the mistaken belief it will give them strong bones. By doing this we are condemning them to hardening of the arteries later in life, hypothyroidism, hypoadrenalism and even obesity. We can all give thanks to the milk industry for that lie.

The government, our research institutions and most of all, our doctors, should have instantly grasped this simple biochemical truth: Too much calcium causes an imbalance of minerals in the body. This leads to an accumulation of calcium in the tissues. This calcium excess not only causes huge changes in our intercellular (between the cells) metabolism, but it also leads to calcium deposits in the intracellular (inside the cell) spaces. These calcium deposits form gravel-like plaque throughout our arteries, kidney stones, gallstones and joint deterioration.

Yes, we do need calcium. Calcium is still important, but most of us get far too much of it. This imbalance is leading to the need to take more medications in order to treat the mineral deficiency-related diseases caused by these mineral imbalances. This includes increases in all diseases of aging, cancer, stroke, Type 2 diabetes, obesity, metabolic syndrome, Type 2 hypothyroidism, depression, anxiety, insomnia, migraines, circulatory diseases, hypertension, immune compromise and more.

What are we doing? We are slowly turning ourselves into concrete statues.

Why have we been victimized by this illogical thinking? Is it false and unscrupulous advertising, a vast conspiracy, or special interest lobbying groups and/or government complacency? We have no answers to these important questions, but our current national state of health is living (or perhaps dying) proof that this has happened to our collective psyche. The proof is in the pudding. We think rational and intellectually honest humans can deduce the truth and realize the error of the "get your calcium" message.

From Dr. Thompson

Over the last 13 years, I have continually been faced with The Calcium Lie. Lay folks can be forgiven for their ignorance of biochemistry, but it is appalling to encounter physicians and dieticians who hold the same disastrous misconception. In fact, I've repeatedly encountered doctors who tell me they are going to continue to recommend calcium to their patients, even after they are reminded of the basic biochemistry of our bodies. They doggedly go back to what they want to believe. This is what the drug company-sponsored research, public advertising and the dairy industry have preached to us with almost a religious fervor. This is programming personified, intellectual dishonesty or just downright ignorance. Could these so-called protectors of our health be practicing a religion, not a science? To ignore these basic facts, after one is made aware of them, is certainly intellectual dishonesty.

The average physician has taken at least four six-hour courses in chemistry in the process of a medical education. This is sufficient for every single one of them to understand far more than the essentials of biochemistry and human physiology. But for some reason, doctors choose to be programmed, to quit thinking, to conveniently "forget" or simply not to absorb these scientific truths. Could it be that their own mineral deficiencies have affected their thought processes or their backbones?

Of course, I'm being a little facetious here, but The Calcium Lie is the result of selective and misleading advertising that has deceived our country and our medical professionals. The cost of The Calcium Lie has been enormous. It has cost us our health and that of the coming generations.

I am amazed at the degree of mineral deficiency in our population. Today, it's worse than ever in our younger populations. Yet, the government still pushes the idea that we all need one to two servings of dairy products or a calcium supplement every day.

Most of us don't need any extra dietary calcium at all! Since dairy products are the major sources of dietary calcium in the Standard American Diet (SAD for short), this opens the dairy industry to suspicion.

When will we ever forget our programming? Please press the "delete" button in your mind, erase the calcium obsession and replace it with the idea that minerals are your body's greatest need, after its need for pure water.

THE SODIUM PUMP

Too much calcium causes the adrenal glands to be suppressed in order for the kidneys to hold on to the necessary magnesium in an attempt to keep these two minerals in balance. This adrenal suppression results in sodium and potassium being continuously excreted into the urine in large amounts draining our intracellular stores of these important minerals, even though our bodies are desperately seeking additional sources of these two essential minerals. These essential minerals are critical to ensure a steady heartbeat so that muscle and nerve fibers will fire when they are needed. They also insure that blood pressure remains stable.

Excess calcium, and the resulting deficiencies in sodium and potassium, causes a failure of the sodium pump with far-reaching consequences. The sodium pump is an enzyme found in the membrane of every cell in the human body.

The sodium pump moves sodium out of cells and potassium into the cells, with the help of a microscopic electrical charge. This same pumping mechanism that moves sodium out of the cells brings glucose, amino acids and other nutrients into every cell in our bodies except fat cells, which are independent of the sodium pump.

It's not hard to imagine, then, what happens when there is not enough sodium to run this pump. The body's ability to get amino acids and glucose into all its cells is severely compromised (except fat cells, which still absorb glucose and continue to grow). This pump failure causes cellular metabolic failures that have long-reaching consequences. Without these amino acids, your body cannot grow and repair itself. Without glucose, your cells have no fuel for energy. That spells a serious problem for you and your body. (More about this in Chapter 4.)

In my practice, I've discovered that the average patient has only 10 to 20% of the normal intracellular sodium content in spite of normal blood tests. That's why I tell them with confidence, based on tissue mineral analysis results, that they are making a big mistake when they boast that they "hardly eat any salt." I call this The Sodium Lie. Almost all of us need more sodium.

GO IONIC

If you are adding supplemental minerals to your regimen, be sure they are ionic minerals. These are the only ones that are water soluble in your water-based body. They are the only ones with an electrical charge, allowing them to participate in chemical reactions that are part of your body's basic metabolism, including in the operation of the sodium pump. (More about this in Chapter 4.)

In the presence of enzymes, ionic minerals allow trillions of chemical reactions to take place in our bodies every second, at a relatively neutral pH of 7.4 and a consistent temperature of 98.6 degrees Fahrenheit.

Ionic minerals are the most plentiful form of minerals found on Earth. They are found in all fresh water, in ground deposits in places where oceans once existed and, of course, in the oceans. All fresh water tables on earth have specific fingerprints of approximately 55 ionic minerals. Fresh water makes its way to the ocean through a wide variety of mineral strata. As our water finds its way to the sea, it continues to pick up minerals, eventually forming the great rivers that empty into our oceans which are the world's "great mixing pot" of all ionic minerals in salt form. These oceans (and sea salt deposits of dried ocean beds), by some miracle, contain a supersaturated solution of all the minerals found in mammals and humans, in the perfect balance and concentrations we need for good health, except sodium. (More about that later.) Sea salt has all the ionic minerals and trace minerals we need for good health.

You may have heard of colloidal minerals. Some misinformed people have pushed them as the be-all and end-all of human nutrition. They are dead wrong. You will be too, if you listen to them.

Think about minerals like iron or copper or even chalk-like calcium. How can you get these heavy molecules into your body?

It's time for another painless biochemistry lesson.

Remember what we said earlier about your body being 72% water? The only way for your body to absorb and use minerals is for them to dissolve in water with an electrical charge, to become ionic. It is simple science. No matter how much a mineral may be mixed, pulverized and powdered, or derived from decayed plant materials (sometimes called colloidal minerals, which, by definition, don't dissolve), there is no way on God's green Earth that your body can use this form of minerals.

These solids and suspensions, no matter how small they are, cannot pass through cell membranes or conduct electricity, so they are of no use to the body.

In fact, colloidal minerals can even be harmful because their mineral residues can end up in between your cells, or in your bloodstream, clogging up things and generally getting in the way. Eventually, these mineral residues become permanently deposited in between the cells, causing inflammation, cell compression, peripheral vascular disease, atherosclerosis, heart disease, and stroke. That's how these substances escalate the disease processes they are touted to treat.

The best example of these harmful mineral supplements is colloidal silver which, over time, will accumulate permanently between your cells, including the skin, causing it to look black or tarnished (the oxidation process of silver). These so-called "nutritional supplements" simply don't dissolve, and their byproducts have to accumulate somewhere.

Since our bodies can't excrete colloidal minerals, they accumulate in between the cells, building up over a lifetime, contributing to all sorts of problems.

Never, ever, take colloidal minerals!

You may also have heard of chelated minerals: They do have their place. These are fine mineral powders, bonded with amino acids, which do allow varied amounts of absorption. Chelated minerals can be important where a deficiency has been identified and needs to be corrected. Routinely taking vitamins or supplements which contain chelated minerals, however, may cause problems if those specific minerals are already in excess in the body, so you still need to have a hair tissue mineral analysis to be sure they contain what you need and won't create excesses. Any mineral can be dangerous if it is taken in excess.

Did you ever notice that your sweat and your tears taste like salt? We lose salty minerals through our sweat and our urine every day. (Don't taste it, please!) Therefore, we clearly need to replace our mineral supply daily.

Replace your lost minerals with ionic (salt form) minerals and find your way back to health.

LONG-LIVED CULTURES

So what's the evidence for these mineral truths?

Aside from the logic of basic biochemistry that my seventh grader and certainly any college freshman can assimilate, we offer the proof of the longest-lived cultures on earth.

There are many similarities between these seemingly diverse cultures, from the Tibetans in China's northeast plateau to the Hunzas in Pakistan, the Titicacans of Peru's Andes Mountains, the Vilacamba of the Ecuadorean Andes and the Russian Georgians and their sister cultures, the Abkhazians, Azerbaijanis and the Armenians of the Caucasus mountains as far as northern Turkey.

The longevity in these simple cultures is a strong indicator of the value of minerals from natural salts, either from the seas or from the salt mines that mark the remains of ancient seas. It's something our society should reconsider. Industrialization clearly isn't always progress.

The modern-day Okinawans are another remarkable example of long life, according to the Okinawa Centenarian Study. The Japanese live longer than anyone else, and Okinawans live longer than anyone else in Japan.

The Japanese government says 457 Okinawans are at least 100 years old. That is 34.7 centenarians for every 100,000 islanders, the highest ratio in the world. The United States has about 10 centenarians for every 100,000 people—less than one third of the number of really old folks as in Okinawa. Life expectancy is 81.2 years on Okinawa, longest in the world. New figures show that the average Okinawan woman lives to 86 and the average man to 78.

Okinawans don't just live longer, they live better, says a 2002 article in USA Today. "According to recent studies, the elderly here appear to have far lower rates of dementia than their U.S. counterparts and suffer less than half

MORTALITY RATES IN LONG-LIVED POPULATIONS

				Age Adjusted Death Rates (per 100,000 people)			
Rank*	**Location**	**Life Expectancy**	**Eating Pattern**	**CHD****	**Cancer**	**Stroke**	**All Causes**
1	Okinawa	81.2	East-West	18	97	35	335
2	Japan	79.9	Asian	22	106	45	364
3	Hong Kong	79.1	Asian	40	126	40	393
4	Sweden	79.0	Nordic	102	108	38	435
8	Italy	78.3	Mediterranean	55	135	49	459
10	Greece	78.1	Mediterranean	55	109	70	449
18	USA	76.8	American	100	132	28	520

* Average life expectancy world rank

** Coronary Heart Disease

Sources: World Health Organization 1996; Japan Ministry of Health and Welfare 1996

the risk for hip fractures. Some Okinawan centenarians even claim they are still having sex. Researchers aren't so sure about that."

All of these long-lived people are from comparatively primitive agrarian cultures. Most of them live at high elevations and habitually eat large quantities of salt from mined salt from local deposits of the long-dried beds of ancient seas. In recent years, the Okinawans have perfected salt-drying techniques that have given birth to a thriving natural sea-salt industry. These cultures also engage in hard physical labor, eat a comparatively low-calorie diet and walk many miles every day, all of which certainly contribute to their longevity.

The U.S. ranks 18th in the world in longevity, according to the World Health Organization. That's not a high recommendation considering the technology we have available. It's interesting to note that the countries with the greatest life expectancies all have diets high in seafood, seaweed and, by extrapolation, minerals from the sea.

Want another little bit of proof? This study came through just as we were writing this chapter in early 2008:

Calcium supplements may boost risk of heart attack in older women, study suggests.

Reuters (1/16/08) reports that taking calcium supplements to maintain bone strength "may boost the risk of heart attack in older women," according to a study detailed in the British Medical Journal. A team of researchers led by Ian Reid, M.D., of the University of Auckland, looked at 1,471 healthy post-menopausal women, average age 74. The researchers gave 732 of the participants a daily calcium supplement, while 739 were given a placebo. Participants were followed for five years.

During the follow-up period, "31 women on supplements ha[d] 36 heart attacks compared to 21 women on placebo having 22 heart attacks during the follow-up period," according to WebMD (1/16, Doheny). The researchers found that the risk of a heart attack was about 1.5 times greater for those in the supplement group, but the link did not reach statistical significance. Dr. Reid speculates that the calcium supplements may elevate blood calcium levels and possibly speed calcification in blood vessels, which is known to predict the rates of vascular problems such as heart attack."

Hmmm. Maybe medical science is beginning to catch on. All we can say is, "It's about time."

POINTS TO REMEMBER

- Bones are not made of calcium, they are made of many minerals. Almost all of us get too much calcium since it is added to many food products.
- Anything we put in our bodies must be water soluble to be absorbed and utilized.
- Using refined table salt leaves valuable minerals and trace minerals out of our diet. We need more than iodized salt and calcium for good health and strong bones.
- Our foods don't contain the minerals they once did because of minerally depleted soil and lack of vine ripening.
- Calcium excess causes the presence of calcification, concretions, or gravel-like calcium deposits in arteries, joints, kidneys and gallbladder, leading to a variety of health problems, including stones, plaque and hardening of the arteries.
- Eating unrefined rock salt from the sea or from land-based salt beds, and taking ionic supplements made from unrefined salt will help you restore your mineral balance.

CHAPTER 2

The Calcium Myth

THIS CRAZY BELIEF SYSTEM EMBRACING The Big Lie about calcium and bones has taken on the fervor of a religion. It's a really dogmatic religion that allows no deviation. The sadly erroneous doctrine says that bones are made of calcium and that calcium builds strong bones. Maybe it's even become a cult.

We're not sure about the origins of this strange and scientifically void idea, but it has somehow made itself part of our collective consciousness. Scientists, nutritionists and medical professionals who are reminded of the basic science that bones are composed of 12 minerals and many more trace minerals, get some kind of convenient amnesia a day, a week, or even a month later, and revert to this strangely insinuated belief system. Our bones are in fact, the storehouse of all the minerals our bodies need.

Medical professionals, in particular, seem to believe everything drug companies say, basic biochemistry and significant medical studies be damned. They won't budge from these illogical and unscientific belief systems.

Where did the sacred cow calcium come from? You're on the right track if you focused on the "sacred cow." Generations of Americans have been programmed to believe that milk builds strong bones and teeth because of its abundant calcium content. We've known for at least 34 years that this was patently false. The U.S. government even validated the dangers of milk, but old ideas die hard.

In 1974, the Federal Trade Commission forced the California Milk Producers Advisory Board and its advertising agency to stop its "false, misleading and deceptive advertising campaign" called "Everybody needs milk." Undaunted, the industry switched gears and launched a new advertising campaign entitled, "Milk has something for everybody." Over time, the advertising buzz morphed to the comparatively innocuous celebrity mustachioed, "Got milk?", intended to trigger our memories of the wonders of milk consumption for strong bones.

In fact, all of this is patently false and the research proves it.

Such scientific luminaries as Walter Willett, PhD., Chairman of the Department of Nutrition at the Harvard School of Public Health, and T. Colin Campbell, Professor Emeritus of Nutritional Biochemistry at Cornell University, say their research shows that boosting your calcium intake to the currently recommended levels will not prevent fractures and suggested it might, in fact, weaken bones. Willett, who co-authored The Nurses' Health Study, one of the largest investigations ever into the risk factors for major chronic diseases in 122,000 women, found that women with the highest calcium consumption from dairy products actually had substantially more fractures than women who drank less milk.

We've got a lot more to say in future chapters about milk and the industry's ongoing efforts to keep us believing The Calcium Lie. This problem, unfortunately, has developed long coat tails. The Calcium Lie has become so imbedded into our belief systems about healthy food that calcium is now added to many foods, and advertising entices us to buy these "enriched" products. Now we find calcium added to soy milk, orange juice, baby food, cereals, pasta and, yeeks—imagine this—a genetically modified carrot that contains calcium! It's not nice to fool with Mother Nature. Be meticulous in your label reading and avoid the "calcium-enriched foods."

We think our readers are smarter than that. We've said it before and we'll say it again: BONES ARE MADE OF MINERALS. Yes, one of those minerals is calcium, and yes, calcium is also important, but we create a grave imbalance in the body if we get too much calcium in a misguided effort to build strong bones. **Remember: Calcium hardens concrete and it hardens all sorts of "stuff" in your body, too.**

BONES AREN'T MADE OF CALCIUM

Here's what bones are made of:

- Calcium
- Potassium
- Magnesium
- Manganese
- Silica
- Iron
- Zinc
- Selenium
- Boron
- Phosphorus
- Sulfur
- Chromium

And traces of many other minerals

That's what bones are made of. Not snakes and snails or puppy dogs' tails, and definitely not just calcium. Let's stick with the science. Any sensible person can see that if we want strong bones, we need to keep all of these minerals in our bones and in balance. We deplete our stores on a daily basis, and we need to replace them all every day. Replacing just one mineral creates an imbalance that has a cascading effect we'll talk about later in this chapter.

Is there a way to press the "delete" button and rid our minds once and for all of the misconception about calcium and bones? We'd like to think this is possible, but we know it will take a conscious effort for all of us to change our thought patterns and remember this truth from now on.

WHO'S WINNING?

This collective amnesia makes us wonder how many other erroneous misconceptions have been foisted on us by who-knows-who. It is amazing how false advertising used to sell a product can lead to a lie becoming a belief system.

No, we're not conspiracy theorists. We're not the kind of people who see the devil behind every bush. It is strange, however, that these erroneous beliefs are so pervasive and so dogmatically held, not only by the general public, but by doctors, nutritionists and other health care professionals who have the tools to know better.

It's also "coincidental" that the big pharmaceutical companies rake in billions upon billions of dollars a year treating the diseases caused by excess calcium in the human body. Big Pharma isn't interested in selling calcium supplements, or at least that's not the major thrust. But pharmaceutical companies are making a fortune from drugs used to treat the diseases that result from calcium excess. We're not making accusations, we're just pointing out the basic facts.

Here they are:

CARDIOVASCULAR DISEASE

Heart disease is the Number 1 killer in the United States. In fact, it is the biggest killer in the Western world. Common prescription drugs used to prevent and treat hardening of the arteries, literally caused by calcification or excessive amounts of calcium in the arteries (also called calcific plaque—there's a clue), include the statin drugs like Lipitor, Zocor and Crestor.

Unfortunately, doctors and patients have been led to believe that cholesterol is the problem. More than 25 million prescriptions have been written for these drugs worldwide and 60% of all heart attack survivors are taking the drugs on the erroneous belief that statins will prevent another heart attack. In fact, despite the massive quantity of these expensive prescription drugs dispensed around the world, the rate of heart attacks has remained unchanged over the last 20 years. Yet the drug companies are raking in $20 billion a year on these drugs.

A recent study has even shown that Crestor, one of the top-selling statin drugs, was found to have almost no effect in preventing heart attacks during a two-year study, in spite of the billions of dollars spent on the therapy. Another report showed that for every 100 patients on statin drugs, only 2 to 4 heart attacks might be prevented. Side effects of these drugs include memory loss, liver damage and failure. Studies that showed serious risks of liver damage from statins were never published by the drugs' manufacturers. Included in the statin risks are: muscle damage (2.8 times higher with Crestor; at least 7 people have died) and kidney failure (found to be 75 times higher with Crestor than with the other statin drugs) and illegally delayed reports of serious adverse side effects by the Crestor manufacturer AstraZeneca, which spent over a billion dollars on marketing this drug alone. And yet the FDA continues to allow the use of these drugs with mere increased warnings to doctors. How about the patients? Who is warning them?

HYPERTENSION

Another case in point: a class of drugs called, interestingly, calcium channel blockers. These drugs are meant to combat hypertension or high blood pressure by blocking calcium's role in contracting muscles in the heart and arteries and, relaxing muscles, thus directly lowering blood pressure. Of course, if there were no excess calcium in the body in the first place, these drugs would not be necessary. For nearly eight years now, we have known that these drugs are dangerous since a paper was presented at the European Cardiology Society blaming the calcium channel blockers for causing 85,000 avoidable heart attacks and cases of heart failure each year. If the excess calcium doesn't get into the cells or intracellular spaces, it gets deposited in the arteries. But these drugs remain among the most popular drugs for heart disease, prescribed for 28 million people around the world, 12.7 million of them in the United

States. And they net the drug companies at least $3.2 billion a year from American sales alone (2004 figures).

These are just two of an enormous number of prescription drugs used to treat the effects of excessive amounts of calcium in the arteries. You can extrapolate the numbers for yourself. The profits are mind boggling. And they just treat the symptoms: They don't get you better and they probably make you worse.

OBESITY

Yes, you read it right. Excess calcium in the human body leads to obesity. We'll go into the details in Chapter 5, but for now, think of a body starved for minerals and the other nutrients that those minerals allow your body to absorb and use. This may seem like a stretch of logic, but we assure you, a fat body is literally starving for the nutrients it needs, so it puts out signals that create cravings in an attempt to get you to eat something that will nourish it. Now we know most of us don't get cravings for spinach or salmon. This desperate attempt to find nourishment causes us to crave sugary, salty and fatty foods that are so destructive to our health. Worst of all, it sets up a vicious cycle of cravings. The failure to satisfy those cravings leads to increasingly urgent signals that our brains misinterpret and stimulate us to unhealthy eating. Sometimes this can also lead to other compulsive and addictive behaviors.

Now think of the diet industry. We're talking about over-the-counter diet drugs, the ubiquitous ads for diet plans and supplements with calcium added that invade our airwaves constantly. Of course, there are also the prescription drugs and surgeries that promise to help us lose weight and keep it off, at a very high cost, and I'm not just talking about your pocketbook.

Interestingly, the average diet drink consumer, thinking that avoiding sugar will help control weight, actually increases the risk of obesity (and Type 2 diabetes) for every can of diet soft drinks consumed, substantially more than those who drink regular sugared soft drinks. For example, drinking one to two cans of diet soft drinks a day increases your risk of obesity by 54.5% as opposed to the increased risk of a comparatively small 32.8% if you drink 1-2 cans of sugared soft drinks daily. Neither is good, but you can see the difference. These numbers from a University of Texas study were presented to the staid American Diabetes Association in 2005. Yet there has not been an ADA statement to date condemning the widespread use of diet soft drinks by diabetics. So who gains here? We think you're getting the picture.

Jenny Craig, just one popular prepared foods diet plan, reported sales of over $400 million in 2006. The diet business reportedly generates about $40 billion a year in income just for over-the counter food plans.

That doesn't even begin to touch the proceeds of prescription diet drugs and surgeries, or the multitudinous and well-documented health conditions related to obesity.

TYPE 2 DIABETES

Whoa! This is a big bonanza for Big Pharma. Not only do the drugs to treat diabetes bring in big bucks, there are all those drugs used to treat the heart disease, obesity, kidney and eye diseases that almost inevitably accompany diabetes, just to name a few.

We're just touching the tip of the iceberg here, but just consider this: 2006 sales of a newer class of drugs for treating Type 2 diabetes called glitazones (brand names Avandia and Actos) were well over $6 billion, despite studies that go back as far as 1999 suggesting that these drugs increase the risk of heart attack in an already heart-attack prone diabetic population.

There are several more drugs commonly used to treat Type 2 diabetes, all of them quite profitable for their manufacturers. In their annual reports, drug manufacturers have crowed about the double digit increase in sales over the past few years. Obviously, there is a lot more money to be made in the treatment of diabetes than in prevention.

Treating Type 2 diabetes can be simpler, safer, cheaper and almost completely effective. Through nutrition, I have successfully eliminated Type 2 diabetes in more than 80 adult patients and completely eliminated gestational diabetes in 100% of my pregnant patients (see Chapter 6).

HYPOTHYROIDISM

One drug manufacturer boasted that more than six million people around the world use its thyroid hormones and another reported 2005 sales of a comparatively paltry $500 million. We will discuss the role of calcium in the development of Type 2 hypothyroidism (thyroid hormone resistance) in Chapter 5, but for now, we'll tell you that excess calcium causes metabolic failures and

Joe R's Story

Joe R was a healthy middle-aged man who exercised regularly, ate fairly healthy food and was at his ideal body weight. He thought he was in great shape. Unfortunately, he had become somewhat of a diet soft drink addict in the past few years, drinking five or six cans of liquid death a day.

Now, Joe knew that diabetes ran in his family. His father, an aunt and a sister had diabetes, but he thought it would never happen to him. After all, he told me, he watched his diet and exercised, so he was safe. Right? Wrong. When Joe was scheduled for routine knee surgery back in 1997, pre-operative blood tests showed he had an elevated fasting blood sugar of 128. That's enough to diagnose insulin resistance and many doctors consider it means the patient has full-blown Type 2 diabetes.

Within 10 months, Joe was showing all the classic signs of Type 2 diabetes. He had lost 25 pounds without trying, and he wasn't happy about it. He was running to the bathroom 15 times a day, the result of a raging thirst that he never seemed to be able to quench. Simple blood tests showed his fasting blood sugar levels were in the danger zone at 150-200 and 250-350 after eating.

We did a hair tissue mineral analysis (HTMA) and the results were surprising: Joe had very low chromium levels, which I attributed to his diet soft drink obsession. We know that NutraSweet (aspartame) in soft drinks depletes chromium, among other things.

I started Joe on a variety of simple supplements and minerals, including mealtime doses of ChromeMate™, a specialized form of chromium that would help replace the depleted chromium stores, improve his ability to process sugars and his ability to use insulin.

Joe's results were really impressive: Within two weeks, all his blood sugars were within the normal range.

He remained on the supplement regimen for the next year and his blood sugars remained normal.

I have followed Joe for more than ten years and he still takes a dramatically reduced number of supplements and his daily minerals to keep his blood sugars at normal levels. We know, because we make sure Joe gets his glucose and insulin tested every three months. His most recent fasting glucose was 99—well within the normal range. I consider that a cure for a disease that is supposedly incurable. Type 2 diabetes is curable, if it's caught early enough. Joe's story and those of over 80 other patients I've treated with this program are all the confirmation I need.

nowhere is this more apparent than in thyroid malfunction. In my practice, nearly 95% of women over the age of 40 exhibit signs of Type 2 hypothyroidism, also known as thyroid hormone resistance. It's not coincidental that virtually every single one of them has excess calcium as determined by their hair tissue mineral analysis (HTMA).

OSTEOARTHRITIS, KIDNEY STONES AND GALL STONES

All of these conditions are the result of excess calcium being dumped in the intercellular spaces in joints, kidneys and gall bladder. Arthritis drugs alone brought in $18 billion in worldwide sales in 2004. Of those, the controversial COX-2 inhibitors like Celebrex and Vioxx brought in close to $7 billion. Fortunately, Vioxx was withdrawn from the market that year after studies showed it dramatically increased the risk of heart attack and stroke. Celebrex and its look-alike, Bextra, remain available with healthy sales although safety questions are still pending.

MIGRAINES

Sales from just one popular migraine drug, Imitrex (sumatriptan succinate) and a related drug, called Imigran, totaled $1.2 billion in 2004. Imitrex's patent will expire in 2009, so it will become a generic drug and will be much cheaper than the $13-plus per pill and close to $60 per injectible cartridge. Its manufacturer, however, has already announced plans to keep sales in the stratosphere by patenting a "new" combination drug that is identical to Imitrex with a just a little added naproxen, which is nothing more than Aleve, an over-the-counter anti-inflammatory. (More about calcium in the cause of neurotransmitter deficiencies and the development of migraines in Chapter 4.)

We think we've gone far enough with these examples to let you know who has the most to gain from our health woes. Yes, we know it sounds cynical and we hope and pray we are wrong, but the circumstantial evidence is certainly damning.

We'll discuss all of the implications of the calcium cascade and sodium pump failure in the coming chapters. For now, if all of this biochemistry threatens to overwhelm you, you need to know that excess calcium in your system can be an underlying factor in a host of deadly health problems.

Too much calcium messes up your entire physiology. Now that doesn't mean you don't need calcium. You do. We all need calcium, but 95% of us don't need anywhere near the amount of calcium we get. Our calcium intake must be in proportion to the intake of other minerals.

It doesn't matter what kind of calcium supplement you take or the hype about so-called "super" forms of calcium like coral calcium. Calcium is calcium and you remember what calcium does, right? Calcium hardens concrete. Remember: Bones are made of minerals. We keep repeating this mantra to help you break the reflexive adherence to The Calcium Lie.

I estimate that we need at least 1500 to 3000 milligrams of sea-salt-derived minerals per day and this is probably conservative. This assumes that you have no deficiencies and no excess calcium, and you are in great health already. In eight years of analyzing mineral status and treating more than 1,000 patients, I have seen only one patient who had no deficiencies at all.

HOW DO YOU KNOW IF YOU HAVE EXCESS CALCIUM?

How can you tell if you have too much calcium in your system? The answer is simple, but the process may not be very simple.

First, you need a test called a tissue mineral analysis. All you'll need to do is clip a small amount of new growth undyed hair, each piece about 1/2 to 3/4 inches long from an average of three spots on your head nearest to the scalp, and send it to your doctor. I recommend that you find a physician trained in this area who is already using TEI (Trace Elements Inc.) lab, the only lab I feel is completely competent to do a proper analysis. To find such doctors, visit our website, www.calciumlie.com.

Your results will give you important information about your intracellular levels of 36 minerals, including calcium, magnesium, sodium and potassium.

The Calcium Cascade

Excess calcium in the human body begins a cascade of negative effects that have enormous adverse consequences to our health. This process cannot be diagnosed with standard blood tests. It requires a reliable, competent lab to conduct a tissue mineral analysis on a correctly collected hair sample you provide. I recommend Trace Elements Inc., the only lab with the correct ratios and databases. You can find information about them in the resources section and through my website, www.calciumlie.com.

Warning: Here comes some more biochemistry. We'll try to keep it as simple and painless as possible.

You have excess calcium in your body

THAT LEADS TO

Calcium seeking more magnesium to try to keep your body in balance

THAT LEADS TO

A relative magnesium deficiency in proportion to calcium that leads to increased muscle tension, and nerve endings firing erratically and other "electrical" functions of the body malfunctioning;

AND

In its need for more magnesium, your body has to suppress adrenal function in order to retain more magnesium to compensate for the high calcium, causing a loss of sodium and potassium in your urine;

THAT LEADS TO

A continual depletion of the sodium and potassium that are stored inside the trillions of cells in your body;

THAT LEADS TO

A loss of the sodium and chloride you need to produce the stomach acid you need to digest protein;

AND

This increases the incidences of heartburn and other digestive disorders, and the use of prescription drugs that have further destructive effects and impede digestion;

AND

Your body gradually loses its ability to digest protein and absorb the essential amino acids that are the building blocks of protein.

ALSO

the sodium depletion leads to failure of the sodium pump, the mechanism by which our bodies get essential amino acids and glucose into our cells, not including fat cells;

FURTHERMORE,

Potassium levels decline dramatically—this leads to thyroid hormone resistance and slowed metabolism;

SO

All cells (except fat cells) become starved for glucose

RESULTING IN

increased cravings for glucose and for minerals leading to more cravings

AND

deficiencies of sodium, potassium, and essential amino acids, and more cravings.

THE END RESULT IS:

Multiple metabolic malfunctions, including, obesity, heart disease, Type 2 hypothyroidism, Type 2 diabetes, anxiety, migraines, depression, hypertension,

and the list goes on and on!

You'll also get information about the most important ratios of minerals, that are critical to your entire metabolism, levels of important trace minerals and levels of toxic minerals. The report includes specific information for each individual on the meaning of the results and recommends specific dietary ways to address imbalances.

The tissue mineral analysis test at this lab is only available through a qualified health care provider, so you'll need a good doctor to guide you through interpreting the test results and developing a treatment regimen. That's the hard part. There simply aren't many doctors who are aware of The Calcium Lie, and fewer still who have any idea what to do about it.

Your insurance company may resist paying for it; however, this is a government-certified lab. I have had patients challenge the non-payment and I'm finding that an increasing percentage of insurance companies are covering the test. It's an investment in your health that is well worth the cost.

From Dr. Thompson

What does this all mean?

Over the past eight years of ordering comprehensive tissue mineral analyses, my experience has shown that more than 90% of my patients have calcium excess, ranging from "significant" to "extreme."

I can only relate this to my medical practice, in which I have treated more than 1,000 patients, but I think this is a fairly typical populace and wouldn't be surprised if these results hold true for most of the population.

This calcium excess seems to be the highest in younger people, while their parents and grandparents have both the calcium excess and serious mineral deficiencies. These results are based on tissue mineral analysis tests conducted by Trace Elements, Inc. (TEI) in Addison, Texas, whose director, Dr. David Watts, PhD, D.C., FACEP, has conducted more than 800,000 tissue mineral profiles over the past 18 years. This company has developed an impressive database showing the relationships between minerals, vitamins, the human metabolism and a wide variety of disease processes. Dr. Watts is one of the few medical professionals who truly understands the dangers of calcium excess and mineral imbalances. I don't have any financial interest in his company, but I wish I did!

Forgive me. I'm passionate about this. The entire Western world is on the brink of a health crisis that we cannot afford. Sadly, it extends to the next generation with increasing health consequences, and at earlier ages, if we don't do something to reverse it now. (See Chapter 6).

Blood tests are not as accurate as the hair tissue mineral analysis (HTMA) because the calcium levels outside the cells can differ greatly from those inside the cells. By analyzing new hair growth we get a picture of the inside of the cells of our largest organ, the skin; we can thereby get an accurate picture of the mineral profile of the inside of the cells of the entire body.

You might begin your search by looking at our website, www.calcium lie.com, where we'll have a list of doctors who can submit and analyze your HTMA. A doctor who is a member of one of these professional societies that are dedicated to open thought processes in medicine may be helpful:

- The American College for Advancement in Medicine, an association of integrative health practitioners: www.acam.org, phone: 949-309-3520.
- The American Academy of Anti-Aging Medicine (A4M), which has doctors worldwide who are dedicated to preventive health: www.worldhealth. net, phone: (773) 528-1000.

I hope the folks at these wonderful organizations will be able to help you find the right doctor.

If not, you'll have to educate your own doctor. Be prepared, this is likely to be a long and difficult process. You can start by providing a copy of this book and perhaps a copy of Chapter 9 entitled "Doctor-to-Doctor: An Impassioned Plea." You can also keep yourself and your doctor up to date by regularly visiting our website: www.calciumlie.com. We'll be posting new information there frequently and we hope to develop a newsletter soon.

Our challenge to other physicians is that they should care more about their patients. They don't really have to know everything; they just have to be willing to listen to their patients and be open to changing their ingrained thought and learning processes.

In addition to getting your hair tissue mineral analysis and following the dietary instructions (more about those in Chapter 8), you'll need to begin taking mineral supplements right away. I always recommend that my patients immediately begin taking a high quality ionic mineral supplement made by Trace Mineral Research or Research Minerals, Inc. They have it in tablet and liquid forms and in regular and an extra potassium "electrolyte formula."

You must know your mineral analysis results to be sure you get the correct supplement. However, either of these is better than none. When in doubt, order the regular formula. I recommend taking at least six of the mineral tablets per day or two teaspoons of the liquid minerals. The liquid tastes nasty, so dilute it slightly into about two ounces of water and "chug" it. Never take it straight.

These supplements do contain calcium and that's OK, because calcium naturally occurs in sea salt. The supplements (and unrefined sea salt) all contain calcium in the perfect proportion with other minerals so it works for you rather than against you. You may also need some other whole food supplements and dietary changes which we'll address in Chapter 8.

POINTS TO REMEMBER

- Bones are not made of calcium. They are made of a dozen or more minerals, all of which are essential to bone strength.
- Calcium supplements, milk and dietary calcium do not produce strong bones. Minerals in proper balance produce strong bones.
- Remember the Calcium Cascade in which excess calcium starts causing adrenal suppression for the body to retain magnesium to compensate. This leads to sodium and potassium loss from our cells and then out through the urine, and an increased proportion of calcium in our cells. Adrenal suppression and hormone resistance results. With the continuous loss of sodium, protein digestion shuts down and potassium loss accelerates. Excess calcium in the cells leads to Type 2 hypothyroidism, also known as thyroid hormone resistance. This creates a host of metabolic problems and failures ranging from heart disease, diabetes and obesity to anxiety, migraines, depression and more.
- Get a reliable hair tissue mineral analysis (HTMA) available through www.calciumlie.com to determine your personal calcium and other essential mineral, trace mineral and toxic mineral levels and information about important ratios of these essential minerals that affect our health and metabolism.
- Take a high quality ionic trace minerals supplement made from unrefined sea salt minus some of the sodium. Adjust your diet as necessary to accommodate your new correct calcium lifestyle.

CHAPTER 3

Osteoporosis, Osteoarthritis and Calcium

SO NOW, YOU'VE GOT IT. Your bones are not made of calcium, so it stands to reason that osteoporosis, osteopenia and general brittle bones are not caused by a lack of calcium. Nor can you strengthen your bones by taking calcium supplements, drinking lots of milk and eating loads of dairy products and calcium-rich and calcium-fortified foods, no matter what you doctor might tell you.

In fact, you may remember from Chapter 2 the Harvard and Cornell research on 122,000 of women who participated in the Nurses' Health Study that showed those who drank the most milk had the highest fracture rates. You now have the knowledge to understand why this is so.

What really causes osteoporosis? If you've read Chapters 1 and 2 carefully, you can probably guess the answer: Osteoporosis is caused by mineral deficiency. It's a loss of the bone structure, the superstructure of your body, because your body doesn't have adequate supplies of all the minerals it needs to build strong bones and, it has too much of one of those minerals: calcium.

Let's take a little closer look at what happens when we become mineral deficient. Bones are the storehouses of minerals for the entire body, so when any of your trillions of bodily processes is in need of a particular mineral, it goes to the bones for what it needs. Think of your bones as a savings account for minerals. The earlier you make deposits (ideally between puberty and age 30), the stronger your bones will be throughout your life. If the needed mineral isn't there, your body may substitute a similar one, but not without consequences.

So, you're right, osteoporosis is not a deficiency of calcium; it's a deficiency of minerals. But osteoporosis is not just a deficiency of minerals in the bones, it's a deficiency of minerals in the entire body.

From about 1,000 patients I've treated in the past eight years and from the database of 800,000 HTMA (hair tissue mineral analyses) conducted by Dr. David Watts over the past 20 years, I can say without reservation that more than 95% of us are mineral deficient and more than 90% of us have too much intracellular calcium.

And it's getting worse. We'll go into the details in Chapter 6 when we talk about pregnancy and childbirth, but here's what you need to know: A baby will be born with an exact fingerprint of its mother's mineral status, so if the mother's mineral status is poor, the baby's will be too. And, as time goes on, everyone's mineral status declines so the picture for each succeeding generation is worse. These shortfalls in our environment, our nutrition and in our lifestyle add up to declining mineral status throughout our lives.

When I look at a teenager's HTMA these days, I find as much as 75% depletion in the total body mineral content and in almost every single case, an excess of calcium that is causing numerous other imbalances and metabolic failures.

Without enough minerals in the right proportions, your body can't make enough of the hydroxyapatite crystals that make up bone matrix and build bone strength. Without adequate minerals, bones are weakened, more prone to injury and unable to supply the rest of the body with minerals needed for other functions.

BONE DENSITY TESTS

These are diagnostic tests for osteoporosis recommended by nearly every doctor for women over 50. However, the American College of Obstetrics and Gynecology (ACOG) has suggested waiting until age 65, unless specific risk factors are identified. This is too late!

We already know that almost everyone's body mineral levels are severely depleted. Research shows us that a significant percentage of the post menopausal bone mineral loss occurs in the first two years after menopause.

Unfortunately, these bone mineral density test results are standardized to compare the bone mineral density to others our own age rather than comparing us to a healthy bone density. As our collective bone density worsens, the averages are lower, but still acceptable to doctors.

Since we know that virtually everyone is mineral deficient, we really should be comparing ourselves to the bones of a 20-year old. Even at that, we really don't know what "normal" levels should be, based upon our current civilization's nutritional and mineral deficits.

Finally, bone mineral density is not called bone calcium density. Remember, bone mineral density is just another way to get a measurement of our total body mineral levels. However, it is less specific and less accurate than tissue mineral levels.

Forgive us a brief aside here: Bones and teeth are composed of the same minerals, so the health of your teeth can be a direct indicator of your bone status.

The National Osteoporosis Foundation (NOF) told us in 2002 that 44 million Americans had compromised bone density (either osteoporosis or osteopenia, low bone density that often leads to fractures). They projected those numbers would increase to 52 million by 2010 and 61 million by 2020. Those increases are staggering! That means in just eight years the experts project nearly a 20% increase in this crippling disease and in 18 years, nearly a 50% increase. Now we know the NOF people mean well when they tell you to take calcium to keep our bones strong. But they're wrong. Dead wrong.

These statistics substantiate the mineral decline and the fact that no matter how much calcium we take, it doesn't make our bones stronger. Bones are made of minerals, calcium is only one mineral. Calcium actually makes bones weaker because it exaggerates our mineral imbalances and deficiencies. Calcium excess causes other minerals to be lost or excreted in the urine.

And by the way, if you think osteoporosis and osteopenia are diseases of elderly women, think again. True, more than 55% of all people over the age of 50 have some form of bone deterioration, but 20% of those sufferers are men. Today, 2 million men have been diagnosed with osteoporosis and 12 million are at risk. Anyone can get it, and more and more of us are getting it every day.

If you stop putting extra calcium in your body and replace all the lost minerals instead, the downstream effects of calcium excess will ease over time and you'll find yourself coming back into balance. Dietary changes and supplements may also be helpful as guided by the HTMA results. If you do this faithfully over time, you'll almost always get relief from current health problems and prevent new ones from developing. Nutritional guidance and reliable supplementation by a health care practitioner well instructed in The Calcium Lie are essential.

I continually stress to my patients how many minerals they need because these essential nutrients cannot be found in today's food supply. A minimum of five or six tablets of sea-salt-derived minerals daily, or two teaspoons of liquid ionic sea-salt-derived trace minerals will just replace what you lose every day, provided you are not pregnant, when you need much more. (See Chapter 6). But those six tablets won't get you ahead of the flood. Depending on the results of their HTMAs, most of my patients need 9 to 15 tablets a day, at least for several months and sometimes for several years, to correct their mineral deficiencies and begin to bring their mineral levels back to normal.

PHARMACEUTICALS FOR OSTEOPOROSIS

There is a class of pharmaceuticals for osteoporosis called biosphosphonates. Sold under brand names like Fosamax, Boniva, Actonel and Reclast, these drugs harden bones and prevent further bone deterioration and fractures in people with osteoporosis by slowing the natural resorption and remodeling process, making the bones super hard.

By doing this, the mineral storehouse gets shut down and more mineral imbalance and deficiencies occur in all the cells of the body, making the mineral bank account continuously overdrawn, with far-reaching consequences, as you'll see in the coming chapters. Cell and bone mineral depletion is actually accelerated if you are using biosphosphonates and minerals are not being adequately replaced.

There is another price to pay for these artificially strengthened bones. There have been no long-term studies on biosphosphonates, but some experts theorize that over time, these super-hardened bones may shatter if they are fractured.

There have been studies that show biosphosphonates can cause a condition called aseptic bone necrosis, in which the blood supply to the bone is interrupted and the bone quite literally dies.

There are documented cases where bone necrosis has killed the bone in the jaw, resulting in teeth falling out. Hyperbaric oxygen treatment may be the only hope for these patients to save their teeth. It's not a pretty picture. Using these drugs will slow bone loss in patients with osteoporosis and osteopenia, but these drugs continually rob the rest of the body's cells of their mineral storehouse, so your mineral needs are continually unmet metabolically. In the long term, biosphosphnates contribute to a vicious cycle of serious health problems.

Biosphosphonates may also cause increased rates of serious atrial fibrillation, a condition in which the heart beats inefficiently and irregularly, raising the risk of blood clots and strokes. In October of 2007, the U.S. Food and Drug Administration announced it would study the problem. There had been no resolution of the issue, first reported in the New England Journal of Medicine, by the time this book was published.

These anti-osteoporotic drugs may be a last resort among people who are already severely compromised in terms of their bone structure, since even supplementation with balanced sea salt-derived ionic minerals alone will not restore this much lost bone. I do prescribe them because of the critical degree of the bone loss in some patients and, there seems to be no better alternative. I always simultaneously recommend, however, as much mineral supplementation as possible and diet changes, guided by the hair tissue mineral analysis results.

Given all these potential problems, prevention is clearly the best route to take. The more physically active you are early in life (in early teens and even before), the lower your risk of osteoporosis. The more weight bearing exercise you do, at any stage in life, the lower your risk. This means walking, running, cross country skiing, tennis, soccer and any of a wide number of activities that keep you on your feet. Recent research shows that it is never too late to start.

Most conventional doctors will want to add calcium to the biosphosphonates and recommend vitamin D supplements as well. We repeat: Don't go there! The chances that you need supplemental calcium are extremely small, and most likely that calcium is going to add to your mineral imbalances and resulting health risks. Vitamin D supplements are not advisable if there is a calcium excess and specifically a calcium/magnesium imbalance.

CALCIUM'S LINK WITH OSTEOARTHRITIS

Joint pain, bone aches, what's the difference? Well, there is a difference, but the underlying problems are closely linked. We're sure you got the answer right this time: Excess calcium and mineral deficiencies. Take a moment to look back at the Calcium Cascade from Chapter 2. When your body tries to hold onto magnesium to protect the muscles and the heart and to compensate for the calcium excess, the adrenal glands are suppressed and sodium and potassium are lost in the urine. These essential mineral levels fall, creating relative calcium excess.

As these ratios keep going up and up and up, they create a downstream ripple effect that can become a flash flood. The adrenal glands are suppressed and the body's cells become resistant to thyroid hormone (Type 2 hypothyroidism) and resistant to adrenal hormones. Think about the effects of calcium building up in places where it doesn't belong, whether it is in excess in the bones, in the arteries as plaque, in the eyes as cataracts, in the cartilage as joint deterioration, in the connective tissues, or the kidneys and the gall bladder as stones.

Now, that excess calcium is building up in your body. Your connective tissues become weakened from inadequate protein digestion and sodium pump failure (see Chapter 4), and vitamin C-complex deficiency (see Chapter 7). Deficiencies and imbalances of other essential minerals and amino acids have impaired the healing process.

Osteocyte cells are responsible for the normal production of bone matrix, but when they lay down new bone over calcium deposits in the joint spaces, we get knobs, protrusions and deformed joints. This process is very complex and many other factors are at play. Calcium excess is the major underlying factor in joint deterioration, regardless of the pathway.

Osteoarthritis is the result of calcium-laden tissues in the joints. When you have too much calcium in the tissue, crystals or gravel begin to form, creating inflammation. Inflammation creates an abnormal healing response and, as this calcium is deposited in your joints, you'll get creaking, grinding and bone spurs (new bone formation in an abnormal location). Increasing joint deformity results.

We know, osteoarthritis is not exclusively caused by "gravel" in the joints or by inflammation. It's also a process of the loss of collagen or soft tissues like cartilage from amino acid deficiencies, vitamin C-complex deficiency, impaired metabolism and impaired collagen production. The result is chronic inflammation and tissue injury because your natural healing response has gone awry. That can put you at risk for other inflammatory health problems also related to calcium excess.

You probably won't be surprised to learn that the loss of collagen is also related to excess calcium, partly because the amino acids that help build these key soft tissues aren't being properly absorbed. (See the Calcium Cascade in Chapter 2 and the discussion of sodium pump failure in Chapter 4.) Collagen itself is a fibrous protein that makes up not only cartilage, but all the connective tissue in your body. Poor protein absorption and vitamin C-complex deficiency directly affect collagen production—and you cannot digest protein without a proper mineral balance.

Your body cannot make collagen without copper in perfect proportions. In order for copper to be present in the correct amounts, your zinc levels must perfectly match it. Too much zinc interferes with the copper needed to keep those soft tissues regenerating perfectly. Remember, (this will make more sense later) we also need a copper-carrying protein, a piece of the vitamin C-complex molecule called tyrosinase, to help us use our bodies' copper supplies efficiently so we can make collagen. So if you can't properly digest those proteins because of mineral deficiency and you can't get that copper into your system or utilize it because of vitamin C-complex deficiency, collagen production suffers. You can see how the cascade of ill-effects continues.

Mineral balance is necessary for the proper absorption of vitamins, amino acids and other nutrients, so once again, vitamins as we know them cannot be used to form joint-stabilizing collagen.

It's the growing mineral imbalance and nutritional deficiencies, not the passing of the years, that make older people more vulnerable to osteoarthritis and other degenerative and inflammatory diseases.

Just remember, we are talking about whole food natural sources of these vitamins, not chemically or even "naturally" derived versions that only contain a part of the complex structure of the whole food nutrients. We won't belabor this right now, but there will be more in Chapter 7.

It's easy to translate this excess calcium to other painful "gravelly" conditions like calcific plaque, cataracts, gallstones and kidney stones as well.

Those calcium crystals can build up in any soft tissue. They are often found in blood vessels, tissues, and organs such as the heart, kidneys, brain, skin, joints, breast, eyes, liver, prostate and ovaries. Not only do these calcium deposits get bigger over time, they also trigger inflammation and other immune responses.

Other recent research shows the link between coronary heart disease, breast arterial calcification and bone mineral density. Calcium deposits in the arteries show the presence of atherosclerosis (commonly known as hardening of the arteries). Breast arterial calcification is often found in women with severe hardening of the arteries.

Abnormal soft tissue calcification happens when calcium binds with phosphate to form hard and bony structures, when calcium crystals accumulate in the wrong places, anywhere but in bones and teeth.

Isn't there calcium in sea salt and in these ionic minerals, too?

Yes, there is calcium in sea salt and in the ionic mineral supplement I recommend. However, that calcium is naturally occurring. What's important is the balance of calcium with other minerals in the rock salt and ionic minerals.

We'll repeat here: Calcium is a very important mineral in our bodies, but too much calcium causes serious health problems and almost all of us have too much intracellular and intercellular calcium. We need calcium in our bodies, but we need it in the proper proportions to other minerals. The vast majority of us aren't getting those minerals in the proper proportions, so we're compromising not only our bones and joints, but our entire well-being.

WHAT TO DO IF YOU'VE BEEN DIAGNOSED WITH OSTEOPOROSIS

Your first step should be to get a hair tissue mineral analysis (HTMA) so you and your doctor will have a complete picture of your mineral status: the most essential mineral levels, toxic elements, and the essential mineral ratios that affect your metabolism, digestion, thyroid, hormones, adrenals, muscles, hemoglobin and overall health. You and your doctor can order HTMA from www.traceelements.com or through my website at www.calciumlie.com. This is the only laboratory I recommend because of its high integrity, long record of excellence, huge data base, personalized service, reporting of essential mineral ratios that other laboratories don't even understand or report, its high level of accuracy and reproducibility. It has the USDA's CLIA certification, assuring its testing standards and results.

The results of the HTMA come with an assessment of the risk of a variety of health problems and dietary recommendations. It goes without saying, follow those dietary recommendations. But the only way—the only way—to improve your bone density is to replace the missing minerals that are responsible for bone fragility.

I'll say at the outset, it is very difficult to increase bone mineral density. Ionic sea-salt-derived trace minerals however, can stop the loss of those essential minerals if we adequately replace them.

It takes time for bone mineral density to increase. Anything over a 1.5% to 2% increase of bone density is highly significant, yet I see at least that much in most patients I treat with ionic trace minerals, and I often see as much as a 5% increase per year.

The proper diet should not be ignored in this equation. Dramatically reducing or eliminating dairy products is probably the first positive step, and depending on your HTMA results, avoiding fatty meats, nuts and certain oils and increasing your intake of unrefined carbohydrates and certain vegetables may also be recommended.

Weight-bearing exercise is also an important element of increasing bone strength. This means walking, running, tennis, strength training or any activity that keeps you on your feet. Gardening is one of Kathleen's favorite weight bearing exercises, although most of us may not think of it that way. You actually get a better workout gardening than you do running—including calorie burn—because you're using all your large muscle groups, including the upper body. I like walking, cross-country skiing, snowshoeing and exercise that creates peace, decreases stress and allows growth in personal relationships.

POINTS TO REMEMBER

- Your body needs at least 12 minerals to build strong bones. Calcium is only one of them.
- My clinical experience shows that at least 95% of us are mineral deficient and have calcium excess. This can actually weaken bones.
- Bone density tests are not very helpful because they are an average for people of your age, and as more and more people get osteopenia and osteoporosis, the lower the averages becomes. You should aim for the bone density of a healthy 20-year old.
- It's easier to prevent bone loss with adequate mineral supplementation, proper diet and exercise, than to try to rebuild lost bone mass.
- A hair tissue mineral analysis (HTMA) test, available through www.calciumlie.com, will give you the information you need to correct mineral imbalances and deficiencies and address the health conditions these imbalances and deficiencies are causing.

CHAPTER 4

Poor Protein Digestion and Sodium Pump Failure

HAVE YOU NOTICED A TOUCH OF HEARTBURN now and then? Depending on your age, heartburn, gas, bloating and constipation may be unwelcome daily companions. Perhaps Tums have a permanent place in your pocket or purse. Maybe you've even gone beyond over-the-counter digestive "aids" and you use a prescription medication like Prevacid, Nexium, Tagamet or Zantac to control your symptoms.

Probably you think of this problem as a minor nuisance. Maybe it's even a fairly major pain in the belly, but it's not serious, is it?

Yes, indeed, heartburn is very serious. It is often the first sign of a major system failure that can lead to a baffling cascade of deadly health problems. Neither you nor your doctors should dismiss heartburn and gastric upsets as "minor."

Fortunately, there is a great deal you can do to stop the downhill health slide that begins with heartburn.

Warning: Here comes some more biochemistry. It's crucial or we would not put it here. We'll make it as simple and painless as possible.

DIGESTIVE DISTRESS CAN LEAD TO SERIOUS TROUBLE

Your doctor probably has told you that you have "acid indigestion" or "heartburn" or perhaps more formally GERD (gastro-esophageal reflux disease), and that it is caused by excess acid production in your stomach. This is another of those nearly unshakeable erroneous belief systems that the medical community and the public seem to have embraced.

It stands to reason that excess acid is splashing up into your esophagus and causing a burning sensation, right?

Wrong! What's really happening is that we cannot properly digest our food because we do not have enough stomach acid, being released at the right time to do the job properly. According to Dr. Jonathan Wright, author of *Why Stomach Acid is Good for You* (Evans, 2001), true acid overproduction is extremely rare. But low acid production, causing just the symptoms of which 44 million of us complain at least once a month, is very common. Wright says stomach acid is essential to digestion and to the absorption of many vital nutrients, including protein and minerals.

So how could excess stomach acid production possibly be responsible for heartburn? It's not.

MEDICAL FACT #1: Stomach acid production declines with age.
MEDICAL FACT #2: Heartburn and GERD increase with age. More than 50% of people over 50 complain of GERD.

Doctors, even highly trained gastroenterologists, don't see the fallacy of putting patients on drugs called proton pump inhibitors that slow or even stop acid production. Worse yet, they don't think about the downstream problems of additional digestive problems. They don't realize that seemingly unrelated diseases like hypertension, depression, anxiety, migraines and insomnia are related to the failure of stomach acid production. These doctors have forgotten their basic medical training.

In order to produce stomach acid (hydrochloric acid), the body needs sodium chloride. Right—salt. Sodium chloride is the body's only source of chloride, the source of hydrochloric acid in the stomach's acid producing cells, called parietal cells. That's why some divine wisdom has created sea salt at 85% sodium chloride and 15% other minerals—exactly what we need in exactly the right proportions.

But decades of medical badgering have caused most of us to rein in our salt intake to the point where the vast majority of my patients are sodium deficient.

Don't be confused. Calcium excess also causes sodium and potassium loss in the urine and a continuous depletion of the intracellular stores of sodium and potassium (remember the Calcium Cascade). Potassium is also essential for the production of stomach acid. Most commonly, however, inadequate salt intake is a major factor.

I suspect that this holds true for almost everyone in the Western world who believes another lie I call "The Sodium Lie." Time and time again, I hear, "I don't use much salt." This is a big mistake! The result: We are losing our digestive abilities and more importantly, we're losing the ability to produce stomach acid correctly, the ability to digest protein, the ability to get amino acids into our cells and the ability to produce protein molecules, neurotransmitters and nitric oxide, leading to a whole host of nutritional related diseases. All because we "cut back on salt." Just like all mammals, we need the salt!

Going back to the calcium cascade, we are reminded that excess calcium causes adrenal suppression so the kidneys can "grab" onto magnesium to balance out the excess calcium. Furthermore, when the adrenal glands are suppressed, there is a continuous loss of sodium and potassium in the urine, draining much-needed sodium and potassium from every cell in our bodies.

The loss of sodium and potassium reduces our ability to produce stomach acid, leading to an inability to digest protein and use the amino acids that are essential to the majority of our body functions.

Now here's another problem: Many people eat Tums like candy when they're experiencing heartburn. What are Tums made of? Calcium. Oh, no!

Calcium Cascade to Impaired Protein Digestion, Amino Acid Deficiency

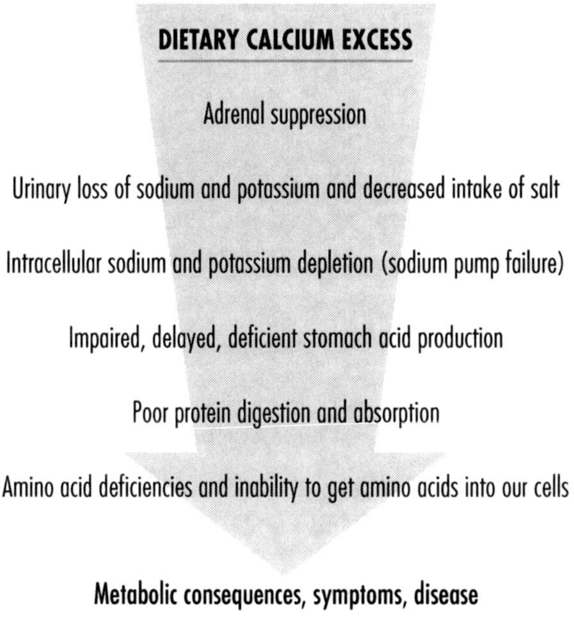

DIETARY CALCIUM EXCESS

Adrenal suppression

Urinary loss of sodium and potassium and decreased intake of salt

Intracellular sodium and potassium depletion (sodium pump failure)

Impaired, delayed, deficient stomach acid production

Poor protein digestion and absorption

Amino acid deficiencies and inability to get amino acids into our cells

Metabolic consequences, symptoms, disease

This means you're getting more calcium that will contribute to your problems exactly when you don't need it. In order for your body to absorb most forms of calcium, you need sufficient stomach acid. Low stomach acid allows those excess calcium molecules to roam around your body, depositing gravel-like residues into places where you don't want them—like in your arteries or joints. You certainly don't want that!

When the stomach receives protein for digestion, it sends a signal to the body to start acid production. I use the analogy of the carburetor start-up system of an old car motor. It is like pumping the gas to try to get the engine started. If the acid doesn't come (like the car not starting), more pumping of the gas pedal is necessary. Eventually, if the engine doesn't start right away, continued pumping of the gas pedal occurs and the carburetor system gets flooded.

Heartburn occurs in much the same way: As with the carburetor and an engine failing to start, too much pumping (stimulation to get the needed acid to digest protein), leads to flooding (too much acid being released all at once because of the overstimulation). This has to occur because there was not enough acid to begin digesting the protein meal when it first arrived in the stomach. The stomach is thus flooded; too much acid is finally released, too late and all at once, so you get heartburn.

Then you "progress" to the need for prescription pharmaceuticals that are designed to halt the production of stomach acid. They work quite effectively, for all practical purposes, shutting down your acid production completely. How can you possibly absorb the nutrients essential to your survival if you cannot digest your food? You can't!

Low stomach acid production causes incomplete digestion. Most importantly, proteins are not broken down into the amino acids we need to fuel trillions of body functions and make protein molecules in all the cells of the body. Minerals are not being absorbed properly or in the optimal ratios so our bodies start to malfunction.

By the way, GERD is not exclusive to older adults. I've seen it in teenagers, especially in obese teens, and even in 10-year olds who invariably have calcium excess.

So what happens when you can't efficiently digest protein and get those crucial amino acids into the cells where they do their work?

The 20 standard amino acids include eight essential amino acids and four semi-essential amino acids, which are needed to help your body to function. Without them, you're in trouble.

Here's a list of amino acids for those who like to delve more deeply into the subject.

AMINO ACIDS			
ESSENTIAL	**SEMI-ESSENTIAL**	**SOMETIMES ESSENTIAL**	**OTHERS**
Isoleucine	Arginine	Glutamine	Alanine
Leucine	Tyrosine	Glycine	Asparagine
Lysine	Cysteine	Proline	Aspartate
Methionine	Histidine	Serine	Glutamate
Phenylalanine			
Threonine			
Tryptophan			
Valine			

Let's talk first about amino acids that help us make neurotransmitters or brain chemicals:

Tryptophan is an essential amino acid, which helps create the feel-good brain chemical, serotonin. If poor protein digestion keeps your body from absorbing and utilizing tryptophan, the results can be depression, migraines, insomnia, anxiety, PMS, seasonal affective disorder (SAD) and even weight gain because of an inability to sense when you have eaten enough. Phenylalanine, a substance found in artificial sweeteners, can interfere with the bioavailability of tryptophan and interfere with serotonin formation, with the same consequences as a deficiency in tryptophan. Tryptophan also makes niacin to help your body rid itself of cholesterol.

5-Hydroxytryptophan (5-HTP) is the food source of tryptophan from which your body makes serotonin, has been used as a treatment for depression, anxiety, insomnia, and migraine headaches.

Melatonin, another neurotransmitter hormone produced from tryptophan, helps regulate sleep cycles. Correction of this neurotransmitter deficiency also relieves sleep disorders and depression, and is helpful as an antioxidant, neutralizing the deterioration of cells and the diseases of aging.

Think of all the drugs used to treat the symptoms of serotonin deficiencies that cause depression and anxiety. You've undoubtedly seen numerous television commercials about Prozac, Paxil, Celexa, Zoloft, Cymbalta and Lexapro to treat depression; Ambien, Lunesta and Sonata to treat insomnia; and Amerge, Frova, Imitrex, Zomig and Maxalt for migraines, to name just a few of the multitude of pharmaceuticals used to treat conditions resulting from serotonin deficiency caused by low tryptophan absorption and utilization.

With about 30 million people in the U.S.—about 8% of the population—showing signs of clinical depression at any given time, there is a multi-billion dollar market for these drugs. In fact, almost all of these sufferers can be treated successfully without these potentially harmful and expensive drugs.

Do you really think your body has a Zoloft or Lunesta or Imitrex deficiency? Not at all. Your body needs more minerals and more minerals in balance. That will result in better protein digestion and more amino acids available to your cells to make the brain chemicals you need to stay mentally healthy. Treat the underlying problem, not the symptoms!

Tyrosine is a semi-essential amino acid necessary for your body to create the anti-stress hormones dopamine and norephinephrine. Tyrosine is also an essential part of the manufacture of the proteins that make insulin receptors, which keep blood sugars steady, and of thyroid hormones that regulate metabolism. It's also a part of the process that creates Coenzyme Q10, a vital part of the body's energy production machinery that also plays a role in creating (good) cholesterol and governing muscle function. It's easy to see the effects of an inability to absorb tyrosine on adrenal function and other biological functions.

Methionine is another essential amino acid essential to the body's metabolism for detoxification, energy production and enzymatic activities, including those that govern digestion, among many other things. Methionine is the spark plug that tells the cells to duplicate themselves perfectly, thereby preventing the cell deterioration that results in aging. If your hair is getting gray or your eyesight is deteriorating, it means your cells are not duplicating themselves as perfectly as they did when you were young. Methionine is a critical element in keeping those cells identical, generation after generation.

Arginine is another amino acid with far-reaching effects. It is necessary for your body to produce nitric oxide, a vasodilator or blood vessel expander that signals your circulatory system that it is time to relax and expand. Without nitric oxide, blood vessels become constricted, blood flow is diminished and high blood pressure or hypertension results. Patients with chest pain are often given nitroglycerin to help relax blood vessels. Arginine has similar results over a longer period of time. Arginine is also important in wound healing, cellular division, immune function, the release of hormones and removal

Jenny's Story

Jenny was only 11 when I first met her. As they sat in my office, Jenny was thin and pale. She certainly looked glum for an 11-year old. Her mom was clearly at the end of her rope.

Jenny had blinding migraine headaches virtually every day for over five years. The situation was so bad, she rarely was able to stay in school past noon. That's not much of a life for a sixth grader who should have been playing soccer, marching in the school band or ice skating in winter. Jenny had become a virtual invalid in this day of "highly advanced" modern medicine.

Her concerned parents had sought the best possible medical attention for Jenny. She had been to every neurologist in the state of Alaska and even to specialized medical clinics in Washington and Minnesota. Despite a battery of every test known to medicine and a medicine chest full of prescription drugs, nothing was helping Jenny.

I recognized that Jenny was suffering from sodium pump failure and tryptophan deficiency. Her body was unable to digest, absorb and utilize the proteins that would help her manufacture serotonin. It wasn't a surprise that she had migraines and perhaps a little depression, too.

I started Jenny on minerals and a regimen of supplements to help her replace her neurotransmitters and ordered a hair tissue mineral analysis (HTMA) that confirmed what I suspected: She had excess calcium and low sodium in her tissues.

But even before the HTMA results came back, Jenny had made a dramatic turnaround. In just four days, her migraines had disappeared! She and her mom both hugged me for joy. There wasn't a dry eye in my office. All this poor little girl needed was a few minerals and the right high quality nutritional supplements.

She was weaned off her medications (you can't stop most of these medications cold turkey without some potentially really terrible results).

Three years later, Jenny is still headache free, as long as she continues to take her minerals and supplements. She is now a happy and well-adjusted teenager who told me on her last visit that she plans to go out for cheerleading.

I learned recently that Jenny's pediatrician had pooh-poohed my treatment and said that Jenny probably "just grew out of her migraines." In four days? Ha! Jenny and her family know better and they're unlikely to trust conventional doctors for a long time to come.

of toxic ammonia from the body. Arginine is also necessary for the synthesis of creatine, which is a substance that helps to supply energy to muscle and nerve cells. Creatine is used commonly to enhance muscle performance (safe up to 3 grams per day) and is used medically as supportive therapy in neuromuscular diseases.

Carnitine, an amino acid found primarily in meat products, is a key component of your body's energy production. Carnitine is like a train that transports fats to the mitochondria, the body's energy furnaces, where the fats are burned as fuel. Carnitine also helps sweep toxins out of the body and helps regulate cholesterol.

Glycine is important for the production of hemoglobin, the oxygen carrying protein molecule in red blood cells. It also combines with cysteine and glutamic acid in the body to form glutathione, an important antioxidant in the body.

Lysine is an amino acid that is an important element of energy production, through a process called methylation. This is a process that allows the donation of "methyl" groups for every organic biochemical reaction in our bodies to take place. It's also important for the formation of collagen for healthy joints and skin.

Serine is important to the activation of many enzymes, another type of bodily "spark plug" that sets off chemical reactions. These enzymes do everything, from digesting food to transporting molecules across cell membranes, so they can be used for energy. It is also important in the formation of numerous substances that sustain brain function. The improper absorption of serine has been implicated in the onset of Type 2 diabetes.

Threonine is an amino acid that is important in protein formation and in the formation of the processes that keep your energy furnaces burning.

Of the other essential amino acids, many have less obviously critical roles and are principally involved in the production of protein molecules to sustain vital biological functions throughout the body.

Other important amino acid molecules include the "non-standard" amino acids that are not found in protein molecules in the body, but act alone to turn on, turn off, carry on, carry out and facilitate biochemical reactions in the body, such as GABA (gamma-aminobutyric acid), glycine and glutamate, important brain chemicals.

We've given you this list of some of the more important amino acids so you can see that a deficiency of any amino acid could have far reaching implications to our health and longevity.

SODIUM PUMP FAILURE

We wish we could tell you that digestive malfunction was the end of this complex biochemical chain that causes health problems but, in truth, it's just the beginning.

Warning: Here's some more biochemistry. Skip this if you like, but it is important.

Excess calcium causes adrenal suppression with a resulting continuous loss of large amounts of sodium and potassium in the urine, even though our bodies are desperately seeking additional sources of these two essential minerals to ensure a steady heartbeat, that muscle and nerve fibers will fire when they are needed, and that blood pressure stays stable.

Excess calcium and the resulting deficiencies in intracellular sodium and potassium cause a failure of the sodium pump, an enzyme found in the membrane of every cell in the human body, with far-reaching consequences.

The sodium pump moves sodium out of cells and potassium into the cells. It creates a negative electrical charge inside the cell that ushers these minerals in and out of the cells. The same pumping mechanism that moves sodium out of the cells brings glucose, amino acids and other nutrients into our cells.

It's not hard to imagine, then, what happens when there is not enough sodium to run this pump, thereby decreasing the body's ability to get amino acids and glucose into all our cells (except fat cells, which still absorb glucose): We get cellular failure that has long-reaching consequences. Without these amino acids, your body cannot grow and repair itself. Without glucose, your body has no fuel for energy. That spells a serious problem for you and your body. (More about this in Chapter 5.)

In my practice, I've discovered that the average patient has only 10 to 20% of the normal intracellular sodium content, in spite of normal blood tests. That's why I tell my patients, with confidence based on tissue mineral analysis results, that they are making a big mistake when they boast that they "hardly eat any salt." I call this The Sodium Lie.

Amino acid deficiency means your body cannot grow and repair itself. Without these essential nutrients, your body will begin to cannibalize itself, sucking proteins from the muscles, brain, nerves and other organ tissues. The immune system is compromised, so an early sign of amino acid deficiency may be vulnerability to infections. Lowered protein levels may also lead to edema, or fluid retention outside the cells, resulting in swollen ankles, hands or face.

Over the long term, those amino acid deficiencies can result in high blood pressure, heart disease, stroke and loss of immune system function. Undoubtedly, there are many more consequences of amino acid deficiencies that have not yet been documented because conventional medicine is so focused on the idea that, in developed countries, most of us consume more protein than we need. Just because we're chowing down on steaks and burgers and getting loads of dietary protein doesn't mean we're able to assimilate the nutrients in the protein.

Medical science doesn't want to believe we could be amino acid deficient when we eat so much protein. Again, we're looking at basic college biochemistry. Science doesn't lie, but humans seem to be very susceptible to unscientific ideas about the biochemical functions of the human body. Doctors (and the rest of us, too) need to take another look at the biochemistry textbooks, apply those basic scientific concepts to our practice of medicine and be sure that we are not practicing it as a religion based on faith in some erroneous concepts, rather than on hard scientific facts.

It also shouldn't be shocking to learn that sodium pump failure has been associated with calcium overload that leads to heart failure, cardiac arrhythmia, hypothyroidism, hypertension (high blood pressure) and kidney failure.

Hypertension is often treated with drugs called "calcium channel blockers, beta blockers, and alpha blockers." All of these are intended to relax constricted blood vessels. Think about this: they're called calcium channel blockers because . . . ? The answer is simple: they're blocking the effects of the excess calcium.

It's time for us to wake up and realize that excess calcium is a major factor in hypertension and heart disease. Worse yet, these calcium channel blockers have numerous side effects, including muscle aches, dizziness, headache, fluid buildup in the legs and feet, constipation, slow heart rate and flushing. In my experience, these side effects are made worse by sodium depletion.

In 1995, a terrible heat wave struck the Midwest and the Northeast, resulting in more than 485 weather-related deaths. The common denominators in every single patient who died was that they were on sodium restricted diets and they were unable to respond to resuscitation attempts.

Apparently, history may have to repeat itself before we wake up. In November of 2007, doctors at the National Institutes of Health convened to discuss further reduction in the recommended daily salt intake. We certainly aren't learning from history.

Now think back to the Calcium Cascade for a moment. Better yet, look through the diagram in Chapter 2.

The adrenal suppression that results from the Calcium Cascade means that sodium and potassium, the exact minerals so desperately needed for the sodium pump to function, are excreted in large amounts through the urine. When the body's stores of sodium and potassium are depleted, the body begins to shut down. The result: lack of energy, cardiac arrhythmia, and thyroid hormone resistance or Type 2 hypothyroidism. The situation has just gotten worse.

Sorry, the bad news isn't over yet.

Amino acids help build protein receptors on the cell walls. And guess what? Insulin receptors are made of protein molecules and minerals. If the amino acid deficiency caused by incomplete digestion of proteins compromises cellular function, the cells have fewer insulin receptors, so the cells can't balance blood glucose. We'll talk about insulin resistance more in Chapter 5, but for now you need to know that insulin resistance leads to Type 2 diabetes and a whole host of increased risks for heart disease, kidney failure, nerve damage, improper wound healing, blindness and more. All of these effects of poor protein digestion, mineral deficiency and imbalance and sodium pump failure add up to big trouble.

PREVENTION AND TREATMENT

It's a really ugly Gordian knot, but one that can be untied with some common sense. All of the illnesses associated with protein digestion failure and sodium pump failure are preventable and treatable. All it takes is basic knowledge of biochemistry and human physiology, and some basic whole food and nutrition.

It's not a deficiency of Paxil or Prozac or Celexa that is causing depression. Depression is caused by an inability to produce the neurotransmitters you need to keep from being depressed. If you just trace back to the beginnings of acid indigestion or the failure to digest and absorb proteins and transport amino acids into the cells and the sodium pump failure, you have the answers to prevention, treatment and elimination of symptoms of many serious diseases including depression and anxiety, obesity, diabetes, migraines, hypertension and hypothyroidism.

If these problems are treated correctly, in almost every case, the disease will disappear. (More about this in Chapter 8)

1. The first thing: Get a hair tissue mineral analysis (HTMA) available through www.calciumlie.com. This will let you know your exact mineral status. Your intracellular sodium, calcium, magnesium and potassium levels are especially important in determining your protein digestion and mineral deficiencies. You'll also get valuable information about your ratios and potentially toxic effects of these and other minerals.

2. Even while you're waiting for your HTMA results, begin to use more unrefined natural sea salt to help bring up your sodium levels. You can fairly safely assume your sodium levels are too low. See the resource section for specific product recommendations or refer to our website, www.calciumlie.com for the latest products available.

3. Begin to wean yourself off proton pump inhibitors and medication designed to lower your acid production. You may need the help of your doctor to do this—and you may get some serious resistance. Stick to your guns. Show your doctor this book and encourage him or her to recall college biochemistry and physiology.

4. Start taking supplements that will help re-train your stomach to produce acids correctly. I recommend Rhyzonate, a form of licorice extract. Chew one every five minutes until you get relief. Over time, this is effective for almost everybody. It absorbs the excess acid harmlessly and still allows for some protein digestion.

5. If you're depressed, but you don't experience heartburn, you probably still have some degree of sodium pump failure. Try this: take extra amino acids to correct the protein digestion deficiency and added 5-HTP (5-hydroxytryptophan) to help re-establish correct neurotransmitter production and bring up your serotonin levels. If you also have anxiety and/or insomnia, additional supplements and corrections may be needed. I also recommend specific testing and replacement of the specific neurotransmitter related amino acid deficiencies.

6. If you have high blood pressure, you'll need to treat as many of underlying problems as possible. Get more arginine into your body to help with nitric

oxide production. A sustained release form is best. I like one called Perfusia (go to www.calciumlie.com for more information). It's also helpful to stop eating foods that contain gluten, which includes nearly all wheat products.

7. Many people with incomplete protein digestion and sodium pump failure also have essential fatty acid deficiencies, so a high quality fish oil product is an important part of the healing process. Eicosamax is the ultra-pure omega 3 product I recommend. Shark liver oil that is exceptionally pure is

Marybeth's Story

Marybeth wasn't unknown to me when I started treating her. She had been a friend and a colleague for quite some time, so I'd observed her over the course of several years. We had shared meals and I'd seen her distress after our families shared a zeal for Mexican food. At 52, she began to pay a heavy price for all that spicy food.

I'd watched her pop Tums over the years and then finally find a doctor who put her on a proton pump inhibitor. There was temporary relief from her intense heartburn, but the heartburn returned and she added Tums to the prescription meds. She was a mess and the first to admit it!

I absolutely hated watching her suffer, but ethics prohibited me from offering help until I was asked.

"Can more medicine help?" she finally asked me.

"No," I answered immediately. "But less medicine will help you a lot."

She was willing to try.

I put her on an acid absorber instead of an acid inhibitor. I gave her a mineral supplement to restore her mineral balance, and encouraged her to use unrefined sea salt liberally in her diet. When Marybeth saw her tissue mineral analysis results and the documentation of her sodium depletion, she became a believer.

Relief didn't come overnight, but in the space of about three months, Marybeth was able to get off all her prescription meds. Over time, we were able to reverse her sodium pump failure and re-train her stomach to produce acid correctly. A year later, Marybeth is still free of prescription meds and heartburn free, unless she really goes overboard with the Mexican food. These days, when our families get together for a meal, we usually opt for something a little kinder to her digestive tract.

I have no doubt that in time, she will be completely free of the digestive symptoms that signaled that my friend was at high risk for serious health problems.

also amazingly effective when used correctly, but is only available in limited amounts. I highly recommend it. (See Chapter 7 or www.calciumlie.com for more information on finding the best supplements.)

POINTS TO REMEMBER

- Heartburn, gas, bloating, constipation and general indigestion are often the first sign of problems related to mineral deficiencies, poor protein digestion and calcium excess.
- Heartburn, also known as GERD (gastro-esophageal reflux disease), is caused by low stomach acid production, not the presence of too much stomach acid.
- When there is insufficient stomach acid, proteins are not properly digested. The result is that amino acids, essential for many body processes, are not absorbed and, therefore, not available for metabolism, growth and repair and other body needs.
- At the same time, intracellular sodium deficiency found in nearly everyone, causes the cellular sodium-potassium pump to fail, depriving the body of essential amino acids, energy producing substances, particularly for heart and muscle function, regulation of blood pressure and firing muscle and nerve fibers.
- The sodium pump failure further impairs the absorption of life-giving amino acids and glucose into all our cells (except fat cells, which continue to absorb glucose independent of the sodium pump and continue to grow).
- Over the long term, those amino acid deficiencies can result in depression, anxiety, migraine headaches, hypothyroidism, metabolic syndrome, high blood pressure, heart disease, stroke and loss of immune system function, increased cancer risk and more.
- Sodium pump failure has been clearly associated with calcium overload that leads to heart disease, hypertension (high blood pressure), kidney failure, insulin resistance and Type 2 diabetes and Type 2 hypothyroidism.

CHAPTER 5

Metabolic Failure

How Excess Calcium Causes Weight Gain, Thyroid and Adrenal Malfunctions, and Type 2 Hypothyroidism

ARE YOU OVERWEIGHT? Is someone you love overweight?

No doubt, your doctor has told you to eat less and exercise more while discreetly adjusting a lab coat to cover a personal paunch. Take a good look. Is your doctor an example of good health? If not, maybe you need a change.

It seems too simple. So you struggle. You faithfully get up at 5 a.m. every day for a morning jog. You try Atkins, South Beach, Jenny Craig and Weight Watchers. You gulp down chromium picolinate, 5-HTP, garcinia cambogia, hoodia, Alli and every fad supplement. You've probably had some success, but for almost all of us, the success is temporary. The weight begins to creep back on until you've regained all you lost and then some.

Why is that? Are we all weak-willed, unable to resist the temptation of the dinner plate? Is our willpower so lacking that we can't even do the basic exercise of pushing away from the dinner table?

No! This answer may surprise you, but we are turning into a fat nation (Generation XL) because we are quite literally starving. That's right: In a time of unparalleled food wealth, we cannot get the nutrients our bodies need to function. Quite literally, our mineral deficiencies and imbalances, especially calcium excess, are leading us to metabolic failures of unprecedented proportions.

We know that sounds like an oxymoron, to be fat but starving, but if you add up what you've learned in the first four chapters of this book, it will all start to make sense.

What are we starving for? You guessed it: Minerals. What are we stuffed with? We're sure you guessed it again: Calcium.

It's a vicious circle: We are starving for the minerals we need, and so we are driven, through cravings to eat more and more food in an effort to get those minerals into our cells where they are essential for literally trillions of metabolic functions. Unfortunately, our foods are low in minerals because of our mineral-poor soil and because few are vine ripened. So we eat more and more. Our metabolisms are slowed because of calcium excess, adrenal suppression and thyroid hormone resistance (Type 2 hypothyroidism). Digestion is impaired; stomach acid is deficient or improperly released. Protein is not fully digested and essential amino acids are not absorbed. Amino acids can't make it into our cells due to sodium pump failure. More cravings are stimulated by amino acid deficiencies and resulting neurotransmitter deficiencies.

It's a terrible, uncontrollable, downward spiral. Since we all know the well-documented risks of being overweight, it all seems so sad to think that we are killing ourselves in a desperate struggle to get the nutrients we need to survive and all the while we are admonished to get our calcium, diet and exercise.

So how does this all work?

Knowing that almost every single American is mineral deficient, it isn't a great leap of logic to think about deficiencies and imbalances in certain minerals causing cravings. Those cravings may be for sugary foods or they may be for salty foods or both.

Sugary food cravings probably mean you are becoming insulin resistant and entering into a state of unhealth called metabolic syndrome in which you have elevated insulin levels, high blood pressure, elevated total cholesterol and triglycerides and obesity. This has sometimes been called "pre-diabetes" because, while your fasting blood sugars may still be within the normal range, you are almost inevitably headed toward full-blown and preventable Type 2 diabetes and all of its side effects, including heart disease, stroke, kidney failure, poor circulation leading to amputations, macular degeneration, retinal hemorrhages leading to blindness and the list goes on and on.

Salty food cravings may also be related to insulin resistance, but these cravings along with cravings for fatty foods are even more directly linked to mineral deficiencies since so many minerals have a salty flavor, including of course, sodium.

Hmmm, salty, fatty food and sugar. . . a Quarter Pounder, fries and a Coke . . . No wonder McDonalds raked in $22.8 billion worldwide in 2007.

Add in all the other fast, fried and super-processed foods that are a regular part of our American diets and a pattern becomes clear.

Food cravings are basically a form of pica, an eating disorder that involves eating non-food items, most commonly dirt, clay, cornstarch, laundry starch, and baking soda. You'll probably be interested to know that as many at 68% of pregnant women develop some form of pica, but it is also fairly common among the rest of the population. This is interesting, since we know that each pregnancy drains 10% or more of a woman's total body mineral supply, so pica is the body's desperate attempt to replace those essential and missing minerals. Mineral supplementation with ionic sea-salt-derived minerals may, in fact, be the most important nutritional choice we can make during pregnancy (See Chapter 6).

Iron supplementation is the most common treatment for pica, so the mainstream medical community seems to have gotten the idea that this eating disorder is the result of the human's insatiable quest for survival. But iron is not the only deficient mineral, and iron deficiency is only a symptom of a greater imbalance in the body's mineral supplies, quite literally the tip of the iceberg. This imbalance is often exaggerated by calcium supplementation, especially in women whose intracellular calcium levels are already excessive.

We're here to tell you that if you exercise like a hamster on the wheel and eat nothing but lettuce for the rest of your life, it will cause no permanent changes unless you treat your underlying metabolic imbalances by balancing and raising your mineral levels. **All meaningful weight loss must involve treating the underlying metabolism.**

Let's back up a little bit and define the metabolic failure that is the link between calcium excess, mineral deficiency, and obesity.

Take a look at the Calcium Cascade in Chapter 2. You'll see the way that calcium excess leads to the failure of the body to respond to insulin to control blood glucose, the failure to produce energy efficiently through glycogen, and most importantly, it leads to the failure of thyroid hormones to be able to stimulate our metabolism.

Low thyroid hormone levels don't cause obesity, but nearly 100% of all obese people in my practice have hypothyroidism, due to calcium excess with thyroid hormone resistance (Type 2 hypothyroidism) and the resulting metabolic failures.

This is what I call a Nutritional Disease Cascade. It goes like this:

NUTRITIONAL DISEASE CASCADE

1. Deficiency develops

Body nutrients (especially minerals) and essential amino acids are depleted, and calcium is in excess in all the cells in the body,

SO

2. Compensation occurs

Your body begins to have some subtle metabolic and biochemical changes, but these are not yet detectable in laboratory blood tests.

THEN,

You develop increasing thyroid hormone resistance, calcium-to-potassium intracellular imbalance, slowed metabolism and adrenal suppression, as your body attempts to hold on to magnesium to balance the high intracellular calcium. Decreased absorption of nutrients in foods occurs and sodium and potassium are continuously lost from your cellular reserves into your urine.

You lose the ability to produce stomach acid, leading to poor protein digestion and sodium pump failure, with a resulting inability to get essential amino acids and glucose into your cells, except fat cells, which are stimulated by the increasing insulin levels and remain independent of the sodium pump. Those fat cells continue to absorb more glucose and grow larger and more numerous all the time.

As insulin sensitivity decreases or resistance develops, more insulin is needed, more fat is produced,

AND

3. Un-compensation occurs

You begin to have slightly elevated triglyceride (blood fat) levels, slightly elevated blood sugars, still minor enough to escape much notice, however, your body has begun to make fat more easily. You gain weight quickly due to the underlying mineral deficiencies and imbalances, thyroid hormone resistance and adrenal hormone resistance, further slowing your metabolism with continued increases in insulin resistance.

You don't know how to treat it, so, you eat less, diet and exercise and your metabolism slows even more. You may, for a short time, maintain the weight or the loss, then you get back on the rollercoaster and gain it all back because your body is still craving the nutrients it needs.

EVENTUALLY

4. Clinical disease develops in two stages

Clinical disease develops, most likely Type 2 diabetes or a neurotransmitter disease like depression and anxiety or migraines. ***In the early stages, it is:***

A. Reversible clinical disease: It can be reversed by rebalancing and raising the mineral levels, lowering the calcium excess, and, possibly extra thyroid hormone.

After two or more years, this becomes:

B. Irreversible clinical disease: The metabolic decline becomes increasingly irreversible, although mineral re-balancing will ease the effects, improve the metabolism, improve the circulation, improve the digestion, decrease the medication requirements, decrease the weight gain and slow the body's decline.

JC's Story

JC came to my office a little shyly. After all, I am a gynecologist, and, as a strapping young man, he clearly felt a little uneasy. What made me feel uncomfortable was not his gender, but the fact that he was carrying 254 pounds on his once-190-pound frame.

Although JC had not yet been diagnosed with Type 2 diabetes, he was clearly insulin resistant and it seemed that a diagnosis of Type 2 diabetes was an inevitable outcome of the metabolic failure that was creeping up on him. In fact, JC's father suffered from severe Type 2 diabetes, and, at 300 pounds, he also had many other medical problems.

JC's HTMA showed significant calcium excess, sodium and potassium deficiency and thyroid hormone resistance nearly 10 times normal. His was a classic case of the Nutritional Disease Cascade. JC made no bones about it: he was frightened. He told me he was committed to making the necessary changes to bring his metabolism back into balance.

We began trace mineral supplementation, diet changes guided by the HTMA which largely involved eliminating dietary calcium from dairy foods and we added some supplements to help lower insulin resistance and correct his mineral imbalances.

His basal body temperatures confirmed what I expected based upon his HTMA results: a diagnosis of hypothyroidism (Type 2) despite normal readings on his blood tests. This was causing his metabolism to slow considerably. He began taking Armour thyroid and gradually increased the dose to correct his metabolism while we were treating the underlying mineral imbalances.

He also began a daily walking program.

Over the next 8 months, JC lost 60 pounds! He was energized and excited on the office visit that confirmed his relatively effortless weight loss. Gradually, we tapered off the thyroid medication and the nutritional supplements to maintenance doses.

JC has remained at his ideal body weight for a year now on a sensible diet that only restricts calcium intake and ensures he gets his ionic sea-salt-derived minerals every day. Better yet, his blood sugars and insulin levels are normal! JC's almost inevitable diabetes was averted.

What a relief for both of us!

METABOLIC FAILURE

The thyroid hormone and adrenal hormone resistance that lead to a slowed metabolic rate is a direct result of the Calcium Cascade from the intracellular calcium excess. It's the inevitable result of sodium pump failure, which we discuss in detail in Chapter 4. Among other things, this sodium pump gets essential amino acids and glucose into all the cells of our bodies—except fat cells, which function in an entirely different way.

Fat cells are actually stimulated to grow by increased insulin levels. Fat cells don't require the sodium pump in order to be able to absorb glucose. Fat cells continue to absorb glucose without sodium, even if your body is sodium depleted. This means these fat cells have a unique ability to absorb glucose without the need for the sodium pump. They are naturally stimulated to absorb increasing amounts of glucose by the increasing insulin levels, which causes fat cells to grow larger and multiply.

When increased insulin levels are present, as in the case of insulin resistance (Type 2 diabetes), weight gain is a huge problem. Fat cells in our bodies are a natural buffer mechanism for absorbing excess glucose.

Insulin resistance leads to higher than normal release of insulin. Too much insulin causes blood sugars to drop after meals leaving you feeling tired and sluggish. The brain soon lacks glucose, its main "food," thereby stimulating your brain's appetite center to try to raise more glucose for your "starving" cells and you eat again to feel better quickly. These low blood sugars frequently lead to the misdiagnosis of hypoglycemia which is nothing more than a treatable early form of insulin resistance which, if untreated, will always go on to develop into Type 2 diabetes.

Unfortunately, fat cells can easily make more fat cells and take up greater amounts of our body's network of blood vessels, putting an increased workload on the heart and contributing to hypertension. Fat cells continue to convert excess sugars into fat. Worse yet, since increased insulin levels prompt them to absorb more glucose, they continue to grow, thereby contributing to a vicious cycle of more insulin resistance and more weight gain.

Drugs and weight loss are not the answer. Treating the underlying mineral imbalance and the insulin resistance clearly can reverse this disease process and return the metabolism to normal. I now have more than 80 Type 2 diabetics in complete remission and thousands of pounds of permanent weight loss in my patients due to the correct treatment of the underlying malfunctioning metabolism.

Hypothyroidism (Type I and Type 2)

The thyroid, a tiny butterfly-shaped gland that straddles your windpipe and weighs less than an ounce, sends signals to every one of the trillions of cells in your body, billions of times every single day. It governs every cellular and bodily function. Without your thyroid, you'd wind down like a child's toy. Eventually, you would die.

Many experts believe that thyroid disease is the most under-diagnosed illness in America. A paper published in the Journal of the American Medical Association nearly 60 years ago asserted that low thyroid function or hypothyroidism is the most common disease of those who enter a doctor's office—and it's the diagnosis doctors most often miss.

I estimate conservatively that 90% of our population has some form of hypothyroidism. Although clinical symptoms are present, they go unrecognized or ignored by doctors, despite patients' complaints. In fact, many people with hypothyroidism have been labeled as hypochondriacs by one or more doctors. Many doctors tell their patients, based on "normal" blood tests alone that their thyroid function is normal and give them a useless "prescription" to diet and exercise.

In my practice, I have found thyroid hormone resistance is beyond epidemic level and it is directly related to excess dietary calcium.

Because hypothyroidism is so common, we're going to spend a fair amount of time with the subject and the easy ways you can address it.

From the Calcium Cascade (Chapter 2), you know there is a connection between excess calcium, mineral deficiency and hypothyroidism. Before we go too far into this subject, I'd like to define two types of hypothyroidism: Type 1, which is the failure of the thyroid glands to produce sufficient quantities of thyroid hormones to keep our body running properly (diagnosed by blood tests), and Type 2, which is thyroid hormone resistance, or the failure of your body to respond properly to the thyroid hormones it has. Type 2 hypothyroidism is diagnosed by clinical symptoms, low basal body temperature and abnormal calcium/potassium ratio on HTMA results. These distinctions are very much akin to Types 1 and 2 diabetes; Type 1 being the failure of the pancreas to produce sufficient insulin to metabolize blood glucose (deficiency of insulin), and Type 2 being the body's inability to use the insulin that is being produced in sufficient or even excess quantities (insulin resistance).

Is hypothyroidism your problem?

Here's a laundry list of the most common symptoms of both types of hypothyroidism. Keep in mind that this is not definitive since other conditions can cause the same symptoms. But if you have more than two of these, it's worth investigating the possibility you have low thyroid hormone function:

- Inappropriate weight gain
- Difficulty losing weight
- Fatigue, lethargy, mid-afternoon energy loss, sleepiness
- Depression
- Constipation
- Restlessness
- Mood swings
- Difficulty concentrating, memory impairment
- Cold hands and feet, cold intolerance
- Coarse, dry hair
- Hair falling out, brittle nails,
- Skin coarse, dry, scaly and thick, decreased perspiration, acne
- Hoarse or gravelly voice, slowed speech
- Puffiness and swelling around eyes and face, wrists or ankles
- Aches and pains in joints, hands and feet, arthritis, gout
- Carpal tunnel syndrome
- Irregular menstrual cycles, ovarian cysts, fibrocystic breasts, PMS
- Low sex drive
- Frequent infections, especially skin problems
- Snoring/sleep apnea

- Shortness of breath and tightness in chest
- Tinnitus (ringing in ears)
- Thinning or complete absence of outer third of eyebrows (Hertoghe Sign)
- Headaches, hypertension, hyporeflexia (diminished reflexes)

Hypothyroidism is incredibly simple to diagnose, but those who suffer from this debilitating condition often spend years looking for a doctor who will confirm the obvious diagnosis. That's because modern medicine has become fixated on blood tests with falsely expanded normal values instead of good patient care and reliable patient histories and ancillary data. Unfortunately, these blood tests often complicate matters and deny treatment to many people because of hard-headedness, ignorance and the practicing of a seriously flawed belief system by our physicians.

Here's how to diagnose hypothyroidism with nearly 100% certainty. You can do it yourself. If you're a woman and still menstruating, do this in the first ten days of your cycle, Day 1 being the day your period starts.

Basal Body Temperature

Get yourself a good oral thermometer (digital is easiest, I recommend the Timex brand which takes only 6 seconds). Put it by your bed when you retire for the night. First thing in the morning, before you get out of bed or move around much, take your temperature. If your average temperature is 97.8 degrees Fahrenheit or less for three consecutive days, it is almost certain your thyroid function is low and your metabolism is slowed. You need an HTMA with a reliable calcium/potassium ratio to make an accurate diagnosis.

Getting a diagnosis

Over the past 30 years, the American Endocrinological Association and independent laboratories have continued to expand the "normal" ranges of TSH (thyroid stimulating hormone, a commonly used marker to determine if a person has low thyroid function) precisely because so much of our population is affected with impaired thyroid function. Laboratories are required to continually readjust their normal values like a bell curve in school. Only a certain percentage is allowed to be reported as abnormal. As the population becomes increasingly abnormal in terms of thyroid hormone production or resistance, the reported number of abnormals has to stay the same, causing a severe under reporting of this increasingly common disease.

Type 1 hypothyroidism is defined by an abnormal lab test, a high TSH (thyroid stimulating hormone) level, with normal ranges from .5 to 5.0 by today's standards. Yet 30% of patients with a TSH over 2.0 have been proven to have thyroid antibodies (autoimmune thyroid disease), indicating they have impaired thyroid function. Doctors typically interpret levels below .5 as hyperthyroidism or overactive thyroid and levels above 5.0 as hypothyroid or underactive thyroid. Yet, in my practice, I have found that treating patients with TSH levels over 2.0 with thyroid hormones and other supplements almost always gives them relief from their symptoms. I've learned over my years of practice that if a treatment works, if there is good scientific evidence for the effectiveness of the treatment, and if it is reliable and reproducible, it deserves consideration.

Type 2 hypothyroidism or thyroid hormone resistance is caused by an intracellular calcium/potassium imbalance in all the cells of the body, caused by far too much calcium and far too little potassium inside these cells, neutralizing the effects of the thyroid hormones that are produced and making them ineffective in governing our bodies' metabolic functions.

For people with Type 2 hypothyroidism, thyroid hormone blood tests may be normal, so doctors won't recognize this syndrome unless they do a hair tissue mineral analysis (HTMA) from a reliable lab reporting intracellular calcium/potassium ratios, plus a careful symptom review and reliable oral basal body temperatures taken three days a month, before ovulation in menstruating women.

In reviewing my records for the past year alone, I found a 99% correlation between a HTMA result showing an elevated ratio of calcium to potassium (above 4.2) and low basal body temperature. This confirms to me that the intracellular calcium/potassium imbalance causes Type 2 hypothyroidism. The degree of resistance can be calculated by dividing the measured ratio by the normal ratio (e.g. a 42.0 calcium to potassium ratio would be 10 times below normal in thyroid function).

Virtually every one of my patients who has a low basal body temperature with an elevated calcium/potassium ratio is put on thyroid hormones. Without exception, they get better. Their energy improves, their skin conditions resolve, their basal body temperatures improve, they warm up and among other things they lose weight. What's more, by showing them their hair tissue mineral analysis and by giving the patients specific dietary and supplement recommendations, we begin to reverse the underlying disease process and eventually eliminate the need for the thyroid medication. I convince them to give up their calcium supplements and dairy products and take ionic mineral supplements to restore their mineral levels and balance. What could be simpler?

This may not be a gold standard randomized, double blind, placebo- controlled study like the drug companies put out at the cost of millions of dollars, but no one will ever pay for a study like that because it would eliminate the need for the prescription drugs that have become the foundation of our society. I have treated over 1,000 patients over the past eight years, however, and have had amazing success in treating the underlying medical problems related to hypothyroidism, including weight gain, acne, cold intolerance, dry skin, constipation, carpal tunnel, tinnitus (ringing in the ears) and many more medical conditions.

Most importantly, this treatment plan works in every compliant patient. It is reliable, scientifically valid, and reproducible. I know without a doubt, it is absolutely true. I have proven it time and again in my practice.

If you are hypothyroid, as diagnosed by low basal body temperature, you'll need thyroid hormone replacement and ionic mineral supplements. Plus you'll need to make some dietary changes that will almost certainly include eliminating dairy products, high-calcium cruciferous vegetables like broccoli, cabbage and cauliflower and increases of potassium-rich foods like asparagus, peas, beans, beets, celery, oranges, dates, plums, raisins, cantaloupe and, in some cases, bananas.

We'll warn you: Your return to health won't be instantaneous. It may take a year or more to begin to get your mineral levels back into balance and rein in the calcium excess, but you'll feel better and better every day along the way.

In my experience of over eight years with reliable HTMA testing, this test has had a greater impact on my patients' health in the short and long term than any other lab test known to medical science. This test has the potential to bring science to nutrition and rational thought to health care practitioners who choose to help their patients get better health.

The mainstream medical community and the holistic medical community have been debating the existence of Type 2 hypothyroidism for more than 30 years, since the development of accurate thyroid hormone blood tests in the early 1970's. Conventional docs insist that you cannot be diagnosed with hypothyroidism unless blood tests confirm it, regardless of your symptoms. The alternative practitioners generally recognized the clinical symptoms, measured the lowered metabolic rate with basal body temperatures and treated the symptoms, without knowing the cause or why they were treating the symptoms, except to attempt to correct them with medication. Unfortunately, these alternative practitioners have been criticized indiscriminately and unjustly.

I'll warn you: If you attempt to talk to your doctor about the possibility you might have Type 2 hypothyroidism, you're likely to get a blank stare. Most doctors have no clue of the existence of this syndrome. If you get this response, give this book to your doctor or, at the very least, copy Chapter 9 (Doctor-to-Doctor) or download it from our website, www.calciumlie.com and pass it on.

Mainstream medicine's bulldog-like determination to diagnose hypothyroidism based on only one criterion has led to The Thyroid Lie, which has left millions to suffer needlessly.

Also, 30% of patients with a TSH (thyroid stimulating hormone) level above 2.0 also have one or another form of autoimmune thyroid disease, sometimes referred to as Hashimoto's thyroiditis. It is not normal to have antibodies against your thyroid gland or its hormone. TSH levels continue to rise because thyroid hormone production is impaired from various nutritional deficiencies of minerals, whole food vitamin C complex, amino acids, and monosaccharides for protein receptors (discussed in Chapter 8) leading to the development of anti-thyroid antibodies. Hashimoto's or autoimmune thyroid disease can also be treated and reversed with appropriate supplementation, in my experience.

Insulin resistance

Insulin resistance, whether it manifests as Type 2 diabetes or as some sort of "pre-diabetes" often called metabolic syndrome, means blood sugar metabolism is impaired. Insulin resistance affects 1 in 4 Americans or about 68 million people. In the coming decades, this horrifying statistic will play havoc with our health as a nation, not only in the physical sense, but in lost productivity and skyrocketing medical costs that are already in the stratosphere.

Insulin resistance has few, if any symptoms. Most people have no idea they have it. However, people with chronic hypoglycemia (low blood sugar) already have insulin resistance. They are merely overcompensating for the blood sugar drops by eating more sugar, setting up a cycle of sugar highs and lows and interim hyperinsulin releases. Insulin resistance is a nutritional deficiency disease, not a hereditary illness as we have been brainwashed to believe. It is our eating habits and, therefore, mineral deficiencies and imbalances that run in families. I refer to this as familial nutrition. It is the pathway to nutritional disease.

If you typically get very tired, cranky or ravenously hungry if a mealtime passes without food, you may have insulin resistance.

Here are the most common symptoms of Type 2 diabetes:

- Extreme thirst
- Excessive urination
- Hunger
- Unintentional weight loss
- Fatigue
- Irritability
- Slow wound healing
- Blurred vision
- Tingling or numbness in hands or feet
- Recurrent infections

How do you know if you have insulin resistance?

In Type 2 (insulin resistant) diabetes, large amounts of "free" insulin circulate through the body, since the cells are unable to use it to balance blood sugars. Since insulin belongs in your cells, excessive amounts of insulin circulating through your bloodstream in proportion to blood sugar levels taken at the same time are the best indicators for diagnosing insulin resistance.

Ask your doctor to test your blood insulin level, along with your glucose level, to determine your G/I (glucose to insulin) ratio. These two tests must be done simultaneously to be meaningful. A low ratio, especially below 7 is very abnormal in my experience and suggests significant insulin resistance.

When most doctors test for diabetes, they check blood glucose levels, not insulin levels. The beauty of knowing your insulin level is that it can help you diagnose insulin resistance long before it actually becomes Type 2 diabetes.

You've no doubt heard that diabetes is not curable. You've heard of the multitude of expensive drugs used to treat it. You've also probably heard that the risk of heart disease that actually kills 2 out of 3 diabetics, not to speak of the risk of kidney failure, blindness and peripheral neuropathy that leads to impaired wound healing and necessitates more amputations than accidents cause.

Insulin resistance is part of the Calcium Cascade. When excess calcium and mineral shortfalls combine with amino acid deficiencies, they lead to the failure of the sodium pump, the body's only means of getting essential amino acids and glucose into all of your cells, except fat cells. These cells (again, except fat cells) become starved for glucose and trigger cravings for more and more sugary foods, setting up another vicious cycle of craving for more sugar, more resistance to the insulin needed to normalize glucose levels and absorption of the excess glucose into wildly reproducing and growing fat cells. It's a downhill slide.

What mainstream medicine refuses to recognize is that the insulin receptors that live on the outer lining of those cells can be regenerated through proper nutrition. At the risk of sounding like a broken record, you know what that means: Increase your intake of sodium through easily absorbable natural sea salt, rock salts, and ionic mineral supplements, and chromium polynicotinate with every meal (sold as ChromeMate™ under many brand names) to resupply the body with the correct form of the essential amino acids and chromium needed to redevelop insulin receptors.

Early on, Type 2 diabetes is treatable and reversible. I'll defend that statement to the death. I have personally treated more than 80 patients with clinically diagnosed Type 2 diabetes of less than two years duration. In every single case, the diabetes was reversed. That's 100%. That's something that rarely happens in the medical world. That's why I'm so sure I am on the right track in terms of the cause and treatment of Type 2 diabetes.

I find that any patient can do this, not by particularly rigorous diet and exercise regimens (although these don't hurt), but by starting the correct mineral replacement and supplementation program and sticking with it. What is amazing is that, over time, the blood glucose levels remain normal and steady, even if the patient misses taking food supplements now and then. Weight returns to normal, energy and healing improve, cancer and heart disease risk are severely reduced and insulin levels decline to normal, over time.

Adrenal insufficiency/suppression

Your adrenal glands, two walnut-sized glands that sit on top of your kidneys, produce hormones that help control heart rate and blood pressure, fight infection, respond to stress, regulate the way your body uses food and many other vital functions. More importantly, the adrenals produce natural steroids that regulate mineral levels in your blood, especially magnesium, sodium and potassium.

No doubt you can see where this is going.

If your body has a calcium excess, the adrenal glands are reducing their function or being suppressed in order for the body to retain the necessary magnesium, to attempt to balance the high calcium levels. This is a normal body response gone awry. When the adrenal hormones called mineralocorticoids are suppressed, sodium and potassium are continually lost in the urine and your body becomes deficient in these critical minerals.

Symptoms of adrenal insufficiency, suppression, exhaustion and impending failure include:

- Headache
- Profound weakness
- Fatigue
- Dry skin
- Slow, sluggish movement
- Loss of appetite
- Unintentional weight loss
- Joint pain
- Abdominal pain
- Nausea
- Vomiting
- Low blood pressure (orthostatic, drops with standing up more than normal)
- Dehydration
- Unusual and excessive sweating on face and/or palms
- Skin rash or lesions
- High fever
- Shaking chills
- Confusion or coma

- Darkening of the skin
- Rapid heart rate
- Rapid breathing
- Flank pain
- Decreased resistance to infection
- Constipation
- Increased allergies

Since most people today believe The Sodium Lie, that they should reduce salt intake to avoid high blood pressure, they become progressively sodium depleted. They begin to suck sodium out of their cells to make up for the deficiency. The loss of sodium from our cells eventually leads to failure of the sodium pump and inability to get amino acids and glucose into our cells (except fat cells), inability to produce stomach acid correctly and poor protein digestion, as we discussed at length in Chapter 4.

Increasing adrenal hormone suppression due to excess calcium leads to:

- Further slowing of the metabolism;
- Inability to cope with stress;
- Adrenal exhaustion from release of increasing amounts of adrenal hormones to try to compensate;
- Lack of sufficient energy production;
- Various mineral and vitamin deficiencies;
- Decreased or diminished immune responses;
- Increased cancer risk;
- Increased infections, especially viral illness, and more.

Adrenal malfunction can have long-reaching emotional consequence, including anxiety, withdrawal and indecision and physical ones as well, including increasing numbers of infections, viral illnesses and increased cancer risk.

How do you know if you have adrenal malfunction?

Adrenal insufficiency or suppression is much more common than conventional medicine acknowledges, and it often goes hand-in-hand with the other metabolic malfunction, insulin resistance and thyroid hormone resistance.

Tissue mineral analysis for calcium/potassium and sodium/magnesium ratios and thyroid function tests along with basal body temperatures are useful in establishing a diagnosis of adrenal insufficiency. Adrenal hormone levels may also be measured with saliva and urine testing.

In HTMA testing, the minerals most often linked with adrenal hormone function are the sodium and the magnesium. The correct ratio of sodium to magnesium has been established to be 4.0. Therefore, if a patient has a ratio of 1.0, the patient would be expected to be four times below normal in adrenal hormone response.

CAT scans or MRIs may actually show calcium deposits in the adrenal glands. That's an interesting confirmation of the problems of excess calcium.

I treat adrenal insufficiency or suppression with increased amounts of sodium (as sea salt) and HTMA-guided nutritional supplements. This helps re-awaken the sodium pump and helps the body to resume the digestion of proteins carrying the essential amino acids that can help restore the adrenal hormone levels and the mineral balance. Of course, I also use ionic trace minerals and I frequently add supplements like DHEA, taurine, tyrosine, iodine, copper, vitamin C complex (not ascorbic acid—see Chapter 7), methyl-donors like MSM and, in some cases, low dose bio-identical cortisol.

POINTS TO REMEMBER

- In the midst of unparalleled food wealth and unprecedented obesity, we as a nation are literally starving for the minerals we need in the proper balance so our bodies can function properly. Re-balancing minerals and reducing insulin resistance, thyroid hormone resistance and adrenal suppression effectively treats obesity and changes metabolism over time.
- Metabolic failure is characterized by Types 1 and 2 hypothyroidism, insulin resistance and adrenal suppression. All of these are downstream results of the failure of the sodium pump and intracellular calcium excess. When mineral deficiencies cause sodium pump failure and prevent the

digestion of protein and the absorption of amino acids, a host of metabolic imbalances take place. These can be corrected with proper supplementation, specific nutritional changes and re-balancing the body's mineral levels.

- Hypothyroidism can be definitively diagnosed by a simple basal body temperature test. If your body temperatures on awakening are consistently low, less than or equal to 97.8 degrees Fahrenheit, treatment with thyroid hormones will almost always produce positive results. Thyroid hormone resistance and Type 2 hypothyroidism is caused by an abnormal intracellular calcium/potassium ratio. It is measurable, reproducible and can accurately predict the degree of thyroid hormone resistance and the need for thyroid hormone supplements. Correcting the calcium/potassium ratio also reverses the disease process leading to this hormone resistance.
- Type 2 diabetes can be treated and reversed in the early stages with mineral and nutritional supplementation.
- Adrenal insufficiency is often diagnosed by excess calcium in the blood or calcium deposits in the adrenal glands themselves. Determining the sodium/magnesium ratio from the HTMA specifically reveals the degree of adrenal hormone resistance or reduced ability of this hormone to do its work. Salivary hormone levels or, even better, urine hormone levels can also be reflective of adrenal hormone deficiencies or suppression. Increasing sodium intake to re-awaken the sodium pump and adding other supplements and, in some cases, hormone supplementation, in addition to dietary changes will almost always reverse the condition over time.

CHAPTER 6

Women's Issues: Pregnancy, Childbirth and Menopause

I'M A GYNECOLOGIST AND OBSTETRICIAN or an ob-gyn in the lingo. I admit, I'm a little mushy when it comes to pregnant ladies and babies. I love them! In more than 30 years of nurturing women through their pregnancies and catching their babies, I have learned wonderful ways to help women stay healthy throughout their pregnancies and to deliver healthy babies.

It breaks my heart to see the lack of nutritional guidance our pregnant patients get from conventional doctors. I have to believe that this lack of proper care comes from ignorance on the part of their doctors (I suffered from it, too, for many years), from lack of nutritional training, intellectual laziness and a propensity to believe the status quo, the drug company reps and, once again, from unfortunate amnesia when it comes to their biochemistry courses during their medical training.

The truth is that when women become pregnant, they become hypervigilant about their health, since that health directly affects their babies. I can say without doubt that this is a medical message that has "gotten through" and this one is to their benefit. While this attention to our health should be in place throughout our lives and, for women, it should be especially a concern when you are planning a pregnancy, we'll take what we can get.

If you are pregnant or planning a pregnancy, pay attention here. This chapter has information vital to your health and your baby's well-being.

Bear with us. We don't mean to be insulting here, but this is important.

Human beings are animals. In fact we are mammals and all mammals have similar physiology.

While I don't agree with much that Joel Wallach says in his 1994 book, *Rare Earths Forbidden Cures* and his later tape and his 1999 book, *Dead Doctors Don't Lie*, Wallach was right on target when he noted that farmers have known for more than 50 years that their animals need unrefined salt in order to remain healthy and to breed without birth defects. Wallach is a veterinarian, not a doctor or a biochemist, which is why he is so wrong about so many things he espouses, especially the use of colloidal minerals. He is a slick salesman, in my opinion, performing the classic bait and switch, telling you about a problem and then selling you something else. Unfortunately, he espouses colloidal minerals, not ionic or salt from minerals.

Yet there is a ring of truth in much of what Wallach says when he proposes that humans can achieve their maximum biological life span through proper nutrition and an adequate supply of vitamins and minerals. To attain a long life, he advises people to take charge of their own health rather than rely on the advice of their physicians, who, in his view, make poor role models in terms of their own health and longevity.

As a boy who grew up on a cattle ranch and studied animal husbandry in college, Wallach knows his stuff about salt on the farm.

He writes, "What's the first thing a farmer or a rancher puts out for his livestock? A big salt block, right? Nobody gives any restriction on a cow, she goes out and has all the salt that she wants."

Any farmer worth his salt (pardon the pun) knows that unrefined salt is essential to the health of his animals and his livelihood. Wallach talks in great depth about the incidence of birth defects on farms where animals do not have free access to salt. Lack of unrefined salt is synonymous with birth defects, miscarriage, organ failure, premature aging and death at a young age.

Salt is so essential to the health of mammals that wild elephants will risk their lives to get to the salt licks in remote caves.

Why do mammals need salt? If you've been paying attention to the first five chapters, you already know the answer: Natural unrefined sea salt or rock salt from ancient sea beds, the type used on most farms, contains all of the minerals we need for survival, in perfect proportions.

In the biological sense, our cells are no different from those of farm animals and wild elephants in their basic biochemistry. We need our salt and all of the minerals it contains, not just iodine or sodium or chloride or calcium.

WHEN YOU'RE PREGNANT . . .

Now think about what happens in a woman's body when she becomes pregnant. She has a little life growing inside her that has needs. That baby will get those needs fulfilled as much as possible, no matter what.

Let's say that the average woman weighs 150 pounds. We know that the human body is approximately 72% water and 28% minerals. Extrapolating that to body weight, that means she is carrying around 42 pounds of minerals—or she should be, if she is completely healthy.

As the baby grows, he or she draws minerals from Mom's body. Over the course of a 265-day pregnancy, the baby takes about four pounds of minerals from the mother or about 10% of her total mineral supply.

Now, babies are not parasites. Biologically they are called saprophytes. This means that, by perhaps some law of survival of future generations, that babies get what they want and need, at the expense of the mother's health if necessary, even in utero. So if the baby needs a mineral that is in short supply in the mother's body, the baby will take it anyway, leaving Mom even shorter on some essential mineral than before. On the other hand, if the mother has an excess of a mineral, for example calcium or copper, that excess will be passed on to the baby as an exact mineral fingerprint of the mother. This is nature's plan for babies to be born with as near a perfect mineral balance as possible.

Every pregnant woman needs major mineral replacement through a high-quality ionic mineral supplement in quantities to bring her mineral levels up to normal before pregnancy and to replace those that are inevitably lost through pregnancy, childbirth and breast feeding.

For every pregnancy, a woman pays a price. Pregnancies that are too close together take an even bigger toll. One of the earliest signs of mineral depletion is dental cavities and broken teeth. I always ask my patients about their teeth and they usually seem a little surprised at the question. A recent rash of cavities is a sure-fire sign that the woman is minerally depleted.

Think back to Chapters 2 and 3. Bones are made of at least 12 different minerals. Bones and teeth have generally the same basic mineral composition, so signs of a breakdown in the teeth are also a sign of mineral deficiency. Listen up, dentists, you can help resolve this problem too!

When we start looking at the impact of a number of illnesses that commonly effect pregnancy, including hypertension, preeclampsia, gestational diabetes and excess weight gain, it becomes clear that these are related to nutritional deficiencies and imbalances that are totally preventable and treatable with supplements and minerals.

Conventional medicine seems to agree that pregnant women need supplements, so a prescription "vitamin" supplement is provided that is little more than calcium, iron and folic acid, a B vitamin (folate) known to help prevent one type of birth defects. (More about birth defects later.) Now, conventional medicine is telling pregnant women that they need calcium to keep their bone density during pregnancy when the baby is drawing on the mother's mineral supply. Duh! It's the mineral supply, not the calcium supply moms need. See, you're already smarter than your doctor! Moms need a complete mineral supplement that they can absorb and use, not just calcium! Patients often tell me their "vitamins" have minerals. Unfortunately, very few supplements have the right minerals or the right kind. They may even have the wrong minerals. If the mother doesn't know her exact needs from a reliable hair tissue mineral analysis (HTMA), she may be making a big mistake. The minerals in her "vitamin" may be the wrong ones for her and her baby and they could actually even increase the mineral imbalances and deficiencies.

The mineral drawdown during pregnancy can cause a host of post-pregnancy problems. What woman hasn't struggled with shedding excess poundage acquired during the pregnancy? Many suffer from post-partum depression. And down the road a few years, 70% of the women who had gestational diabetes will develop Type 2 diabetes.

For the most part, conventional medicine only uses drugs to deal with these problems during pregnancy and afterward. You've read far enough in this book now to know that Type 2 diabetes, Type 2 hypothyroidism, obesity, migraine headaches, insomnia, anxiety and depression are all related to mineral status and that correcting deficiencies and imbalances will treat and prevent these diseases.

It's worth a few paragraphs to discuss gestational diabetes here, since it is such a serious and increasingly common problem that leads to even more serious problems years later.

Doctors fail to diagnose at least 20% of today's cases of gestational diabetes because they have failed to consider the significance of the insulin resistance measurement in accurately diagnosing the problem. Unfortunately, when they do make the diagnosis correctly in the other 80%, they treat gestational diabetes with caloric restriction, insulin and sometimes drugs.

You'll remember in Chapter 5, we talked about a glucose/insulin (G/I) ratio that gives us a definitive diagnosis of Type 2 diabetes, and gestational diabetes as well. Impaired blood glucose tolerance because of insulin resistance is impaired glucose tolerance, whether you're pregnant or not.

The only good thing about gestational diabetes is that it usually goes into remission after the baby is born, although the risk of its return in later years is over 70%, because the underlying problem has not been treated. This underlying problem, insulin resistance, contributes to difficulty with weight loss and often continued weight gain after pregnancy. If the doctor would merely perform an insulin level with every blood glucose test, elevated insulin levels, low glucose/insulin level and insulin resistance can be accurately diagnosed.

Instead of these simple blood tests, conventional doctors merely rely on a blood glucose reading, which is often inaccurate and then they leap to a grueling three-hour glucose tolerance test, leaving out essential information, the G/I ratio. It is important to remember that in the practice of medicine, any abnormal test is more significant than a normal one in most cases. If the blood glucose level is above normal or the G/I ratio is below normal, this is significant in every case and implies insulin resistance. Ask your doctor to perform an insulin level and calculate the G/I ratio every time a glucose level is taken. If this is not done, you risk missing the diagnosis of insulin resistance before it can hurt you or your loved one.

Medical science tells us several things about what happens to a woman after multiple pregnancies:

- If a woman has repeated pregnancies that are less than 2 years apart, her risk of miscarriage and her baby's risk of birth defects increases.
- With each pregnancy, the risk of miscarriage and birth defects increases.
- As a woman ages, her risk of birth defects and miscarriages increases.
- If she has a previous pregnancy affected by a birth defect, her risk of having another is increased.
- If a woman has had more than three miscarriages, her rate of subsequent miscarriage goes up significantly.

All of the above problems of multiple pregnancies are largely due to increased mineral depletion and imbalance.

Miscarriages are also related to mineral deficiencies. Also, it has been shown that over 70% of all miscarriages are related to chromosomal abnormality, which is nearly always associated with birth defects, as well as mental retardation. Almost all other serious birth defects which cause infant death are sporadic, not chromosomal. More than 50% of infant deaths in the

Teresa's Story

I think of Teresa as the candle lady because she always brought a small gift when she came to my office, for me or my wife or my staff. Often she gave us little candles, a thoughtful gesture we don't often see.

Teresa had great difficulty getting pregnant. She had suffered two early miscarriages and, at 38, she was afraid her biological clock was running down. Her HTMA showed a variety of mineral deficiencies and imbalances, and I thought her infertility might be related to her mineral status, so I started her on ionic minerals.

We all rejoiced when, four months later, we confirmed Teresa was pregnant.

Her pregnancy was routine until we got to the 22nd week, about five and one half months, when she began to gain weight rapidly. She had already eliminated dairy products from her diet, so I was concerned she might be showing signs of developing gestational diabetes. I ordered a glucose/insulin screen that wouldn't normally have taken place until six weeks further into her pregnancy.

The results came back as I had suspected: her glucose/insulin ratio was very low. A glucose tolerance test with insulin levels at every increment confirmed the diagnosis: Teresa had gestational diabetes. Needless to say, she was very worried since she had such difficulty conceiving, and she had successfully carried her baby through the most dangerous first trimester.

"What can I do, Dr. Thompson?" she pleaded with me as she dabbed at her eyes with a tissue.

I placed her on gradually increasing levels of ChromeMate™, a patented nicotinic acid-bound form of chromium, with every meal. She also started on 100% whole food vitamins and large amounts of trace minerals. She was testing her fasting blood sugars every morning and two hours after one of her meals, until her glucose readings were within the normal ranges.

It took about three weeks for Teresa to get her ChromeMate™ intake to the place where her sugars were normal. From there, it was smooth sailing. Her weight gain was within the expected amounts and she went on to deliver an 11-pound baby boy with completely normal blood sugars after birth.Teresa's sugars also remained normal after the stress of the delivery.

As an interesting (and sad) aside, several of my fellow doctors and some of the nurses noticed that Teresa's and her baby's blood sugars were perfectly normal after delivery, but none of them asked me how this could be in a mother diagnosed with gestational diabetes or asked what I had done to address the problem. I volunteered the information, explaining the reason for the wonderful outcome for Teresa and her baby, but they just shrugged and dismissed it as an "unexplained" improvement.

The patient went on to lose her pregnancy weight and then some. Baby and Mom are beautifully healthy today and share their story often, but their success usually falls on deaf ears. Maybe the health concerns of pregnant women blind them to possibilities of better health, and they invariably tell Teresa they'll just follow their doctors' order. It's their loss and that of their precious babies.

United States are caused by one of these two factors. Imagine the impact if we merely treated the human animal as well as our farm animals and provided the missing and deficient minerals, not just calcium and assorted other imbalanced chelated minerals as are found in the typical prenatal "vitamins"!

What is the common denominator in all these circumstances? The common denominator in these sad scenarios is that the mother's mineral storehouse has been consistently depleted by her babies and she has not taken the time or the necessary minerals to regain or replace what she has lost. These mineral deficiencies and imbalances get worse with age and are rapidly depleted in pregnancy for all the reasons we have previously discussed: the lack of ionic minerals in our diet.

Imagine a woman who has had five children who potentially would have had her mineral storehouse depleted by 50%! If she's like most women, she would not have started with optimal mineral levels and balance. It's hard to imagine how she could be walking around, much less caring for five kids and doing all the things that modern moms do. Life alone would make her tired, but when you consider the mineral depletion the pregnancies have caused, it's no wonder she has problems with depression, weight, energy, migraines, hormones and mood.

It's also amazing how forgiving and adaptable the human body is. It never ceases to amaze me when I see someone who, on paper, looks like she should be at death's door, and she is actually coping rather well.

These conditions are reversible. Time and time again, I've seen how quickly a woman can regain her mineral stores, her energy, her optimal weight and recover from blood sugar imbalances experienced during pregnancy with a simple regimen of the right minerals, supplements and eating habits guided by her HTMA.

CALCIUM PROBLEMS

There are two common complications of pregnancy that we haven't mentioned yet, which bear some discussion.

The first is pregnancy-induced hypertension or high blood pressure. In Chapter 5, we explained how the Calcium Cascade can lead to sodium pump failure and the process by which that can cause high blood pressure, vascular dysfunction and a shortfall of nitric oxide production that dilates blood vessels. As with many complications of pregnancy, it's best to prevent them rather than to treat them, so getting your minerals and amino acids in balance before a pregnancy is your best bet. However, experts estimate that half of the pregnancies in the U.S. aren't exactly planned. So it's best to be at optimal mineral and nutritional levels all the time.

Another relatively unfamiliar complication is calcification of the placenta. This is caused by excess intracellular calcium. The placenta is a fascinating organ, programmed to be born, serve its purpose of protecting and nourishing the fetus and die in about 9.5 months. Because of its fast forward lifespan, the placenta is a good reflection of general body health. If the placenta starts to harden (just like a hardening artery), the pregnancy is in trouble. If we see a fully mature placenta two, three or even four weeks before term or more, very often the baby isn't getting the nutrients it needs, growth starts to slow and sometimes we even have to deliver the baby early.

A blood pressure drop is standard at about 20 weeks of pregnancy. If that blood pressure drop doesn't occur or if the blood pressure is above normal early in pregnancy, I immediately put the mother on ionic minerals and shark liver oil (high in healthy fats and alkyl glycerols). In every case, for over 12 years now, blood pressure problems have been stopped and the pregnancy continues normally.

Avoiding calcium excess is the best way to prevent both pregnancy induced hypertension and calcification of the placenta. I think every woman who becomes pregnant should have an HTMA (if she hasn't already) and she, like nearly everyone else in the country, needs ionic mineral supplements. In my experience, this treatment pretty much eliminates every hypertension complication in pregnancy. Since I learned about whole food supplements, trace minerals and shark liver oil in 1996, I have not had to deliver a baby early because of hypertension or preeclampsia. Shark liver oil high in alkyl glycerols is my recommended supplement. Other fish oils do not work, or not as well.

THINKING IT THROUGH

Let's think about this for a moment.

We now know that most American adults have only about 10–20% of the intracellular sodium reserves we need, due to calcium excess inside their cells.

That includes women.

So when a woman becomes pregnant, she has only 10% to 20% of the sodium she needs to drive her sodium pump and bring minerals and essential amino acids into her cells.

She then passes on this depleted mineral status to her baby, as she gets more critically nutritionally deficient with each pregnancy.

Perhaps one of the first things that happens is that the baby gets gas and indigestion in the first month of life. Already, the poor little tyke is experiencing protein digestive failure. Maybe the pediatrician even prescribes proton pump inhibitors. You can see where this is going. The Calcium Cascade (Chapter 2) is already taking place in a tiny baby!

What lies ahead for this little one?

We know that kids have poor eating habits today. My heart aches when I see what people feed their kids these days: Comfort foods, fast foods, juice by the gallon, even soft drinks. Wow! No wonder these kids are sick all the time.

Over time, these little ones grow, but not very well. We hear of more and more life-impacting sports injuries in Little Leaguers and increasing allergy problems that indicate severe immune system compromise. I know here in Anchorage, Alaska, the number of children carrying epi-pens to school because of life-threatening allergies has increased by 500% in the last ten years.

By the time a child is in elementary school, she's probably overweight or he has at least one chronic health problem.

The failure of protein digestion and the sodium pump can occur at an astonishingly young age. We know this because we are seeing more and more cases of metabolic failure, like Type 2 diabetes, in young children and teens. Type 2 diabetes was once called Adult Onset Diabetes, but that name has become inaccurate, since so many children and teenagers are being diagnosed these days. Obesity is the common factor among almost every single child with Type 2 diabetes and, even before they become obese, almost all of these children have Type 2 hypothyroidism.

You don't have to re-read the earlier sections of this book to understand how failure to digest protein, sodium pump failure and metabolic dysfunction lead to these problems. This is a national catastrophe of untold proportions. Where once a 50- or 60-year old might be diagnosed with Type 2 diabetes and expect that the terrible diseases that accompany diabetes—like heart disease, kidney failure, vision problems that lead to blindness, circulatory problems that cause poor wound healing and necessitate amputations in 10 or 15 or 20 years, we face a much more grim reality today.

Now think of a 15-year old diagnosed with Type 2 diabetes and with high cholesterol at 21. Fifteen years later, he is only 36 and already suffering from hypertension, morbid obesity and high cholesterol. Think of a 15-year old girl with the same problem and as soon as she has a baby, her mineral status is even further compromised. As teenagers, both of these hypothetical kids suffer from Type 2 hypothyroidism and, by the age of 40, they are in need of heart bypass or gastric bypass surgery. Their life expectancies are dramatically shortened and the quality of what life they have left is severely compromised. This is one of the reasons why experts say that, for the first time in modern history, our children's life expectancies are shorter than our own.

Frightening, isn't it?

I actually find it exasperating, because all of this could quite simply be prevented and treated by increasing and balancing minerals, adding whole food nutritional supplements and making HTMA directed dietary changes.

BIRTH DEFECTS ARE PREVENTABLE

What would you say if I told you that I have a formula that will eliminate more than 50%, if not all, birth defects? It's true and it's based on the same basic biochemistry that any pre-med student must understand to proceed to medical school.

Half of the children born with major birth defects in the U.S. will die within the first six months of life. Statistically, those children with severe birth defects probably have little chance for survival, as sad as it may seem.

Some major birth defects are associated with carried genetic traits. Many other defects are caused by spontaneous chromosome abnormalities, like Down Syndrome. These two types of birth defect-related problems are the most likely to be prevented through aggressive mineral supplementation and balancing.

This is where animal husbandry on the farm has made the greatest strides. A 70% reduction in miscarriage and a 98% reduction in birth defects with mineral supplementation in animals is easy to translate to the human experience. If we eliminate mineral deficiencies and imbalances before conception, 98% of these birth defects would be prevented. This would mean we could reduce infant deaths by more than 50% in as little as one year.

The other half of the children born with major birth defects have chromosome abnormalities and their associated birth defects, and somehow, these pregnancies escape miscarriage and the children go on to be born. It remains unclear as to whether mineral replacement could completely reduce or eliminate these birth tragedies. Again, however, based on animal husbandry data, a reduction of up to 70% could be expected.

There is no intervention in health care history that could have a greater impact on life and death. Neonatal mortality has an impact that goes on for generations. The pain and suffering lasts a lifetime. This is not an expensive fix. We must give our children the healthiest possible start in life. This simple fix would obviously also have a major impact on healthcare expenditures in the US.

If we are smart enough to give our farm animals sea salt to prevent birth defects, why aren't we smart enough to do it for ourselves?

Several years ago, it was recognized that folic acid deficiency was a major factor in neural tube defects, one type of birth defect. The neural tube is a structure present in embryos that eventually develops into the central nervous system. Defects in the neural tube, developed in early pregnancy, can result in a variety of deformities in spine and brain development in children. What followed was a folic acid frenzy. It became a necessity in prenatal vitamins and the government mandated the addition of folic acid to common foods (primarily flours and cereals).

That is all well and good. The Centers for Disease Control and Prevention says that since 1996, when the Food and Drug Administration mandated the folic acid fortification program, the number of neural tube defects has declined by about 25%.

That's excellent, but it's only a tiny part of the picture. It's only one type of birth defect. Only about 2,500 babies are born in the U.S. each year with neural tube defects. About half of those are linked to folic acid deficiency in mothers.

That is about 1% of the babies born with birth defects every year. The March of Dimes estimates there are 120,000 babies born with major birth defects in the U.S. each year. The cause of 70% of those is "unknown" to medical science, but I think we can make a pretty good guess.

I have no problem with the folic acid fortification program, but I think it doesn't go far enough. I firmly believe, and it has been substantiated in my practice, that we could eliminate 98% of birth defects in the United States with a simple trace mineral supplementation program for every women.

It would be even more effective if the supplementation began before the woman became pregnant, maybe even in the teenage years, since the majority of birth defects occur in the first month of pregnancy, often before a woman is even aware she is pregnant. Obviously, there are other factors to consider, since minerals are a nutritional necessity for strong bones and good health. Ongoing supplementation simply makes common sense.

MENOPAUSE

What we have covered in this chapter and the previous chapter applies very well to menopause. It is estimated that as many as 40% of perimenopausal (pre-menopausal) women have low thyroid function that adds to their symptoms when hormones begin to fluctuate as full menopause approaches. I believe this statistic is conservative.

If you think back to the symptoms of Types 1 and 2 hypothyroidism, the fatigue, irritability, insomnia, weight gain, mood and energy swings, and more, these sound remarkably like the symptoms of menopause. That's because the underlying factors of impaired hormone production and impaired hormone function are the same: excess intracellular calcium (remember the Calcium Cascade), incomplete protein digestion, sodium pump failure, and ultimately, clinical symptoms.

In addition, the major female hormones estrogen and progesterone lose their effectiveness when there is a zinc/copper imbalance, which frequently occurs with calcium excess and mineral imbalances or deficiencies. In fact, hormones need minerals in order to do their work, so when minerals are missing or unbalanced, hormones will be out of whack. Add that to the hormonal fluctuations that begin as a woman nears the end of her childbearing years and her hormones start to spike and bottom out in unpredictable ways. You get the picture.

To make matters worse, many menopausal women begin to take more and more calcium supplements because of the widely espoused fear of osteoporosis. We know that by taking these supplements, they are causing their mineral status to become more unbalanced and this further aggravates the Calcium Cascade.

Finally, there are political and pharmaceutical forces afoot that are trying to take away a woman's right to use the only safe hormone replacement therapy, bioidentical hormones. These are the exact same hormones that replace the hormones already naturally occurring in women's bodies with hormones identical to those present before menopause. These are available only by prescription and only from specialized compounding pharmacies, because they are not patentable. They are basically generic. I'm not much of an activist, but this is an outrageous, most blatant effort by drug companies to squelch competition and, if all of us don't fight back, we'll all lose. You can contact your elected officials through the FANS (Freedom of Access to Natural Solutions) website at: www.projectfans.org/law-legislation.cfm.

Never, ever take synthetic or "equine-based" hormones. These are hormones made from the urine of pregnant mares, and they contain estrogens never ever before found in women's bodies. Most notably, these are Premarin (PREgnant MARes' urINe) and Prempro, which contains Premarin and synthetic "progesterone" or progestin (it's actually a testosterone derivative). These drugs have been proven by large studies not only to increase the risk of breast cancer and blood clotting, but they dramatically increase the risk of heart attack, stroke and Alzheimer's disease. Don't do it! Remember, there can be no comparison of these chemicals to bioidentical hormones that naturally exist, safely in women's bodies.

Now here's the zinger: Guess who filed the complaint that may lead to the end of the era of compounding pharmacies and bioidentical hormone replacement? Wyeth Pharmaceuticals, the manufacturer of Premarin and Prempro. That's the same company whose sales suddenly plummeted into the toilet after research proved their products were downright dangerous to women. So far they have lost nearly $1 billion or more in sales.

These were products that had been in use for 50 years, and virtually every doctor had been brainwashed into believing these horse-estrogens would protect women from osteoporosis, heart disease and strokes. The Premarin Lie has probably killed hundreds of thousands of women over the years. And now Wyeth wants to kill the competition, the place where many women have turned for safe hormone replacement. It's an outrage!

Interestingly, Wyeth is doing this in the name of "safety and protecting the public." And they are getting away with it, so far. This company should be ashamed and so should the politicians and FDA bureaucrats who have listened to their lobbying efforts. In my opinion, Wyeth should be banned from selling products related to women's health forever. They care only about money. They have misled enough doctors and patients and caused enough death and heartache already! Worse yet, they have yet to be held accountable.

POINTS TO REMEMBER

- Pregnant women lose approximately 10% of their total mineral supply to their babies.
- Too many pregnancies too close together can severely compromise the mother's health and increase the risk of birth defects from excessive mineral loss.
- Babies are programmed to take the minerals they need, even if the mother can't afford to lose them, because of their own deficiencies and imbalances.
- Babies are born with an exact fingerprint of their mother's mineral status.
- Imbalanced minerals on the part of the mother are passed on to the baby, resulting in mineral imbalances and deficiencies from birth.
- Infants and young children suffer the effects of calcium excess and mineral imbalances and deficiencies. These problems increase throughout a lifetime, due to the lack of ionic minerals in the diet, continued mineral loss and calcium excess in the diet.
- Birth defects can be reduced by over 50%, if not completely eliminated, miscarriage reduced by over 70% and infant death reduced by over 50% with adequate ionic minerals and supplements. These figures are based on more than 50 years of animal data.
- The problems many women experience with menopause are largely attributable to calcium excess, impaired protein digestion, and sodium pump failure. Mineral balancing, nutritional corrections and bioidentical hormones will keep hypothyroidism, weight gain, depression, irritability and insomnia at bay and greatly improve the quality of life of women.
- There is overwhelming biological evidence that bio-identical hormone replacement is not only natural and safe, but it improves the quality of life and reduces breast cancer incidence.

CHAPTER 7

The Vitamin Lie

WE ALL KNOW WE NEED VITAMINS in order to survive. Without minerals, none of these vitamins, sometimes called co-enzymes, can be used by the human body, since minerals are part of the transport system that brings the vitamins into the cells where they are needed.

Minerals are also needed to donate the electrons for all biochemical reactions that vitamins help to take place. Vitamins simply do not work without minerals. Furthermore, vitamins cannot be formed without minerals and trace minerals.

So, not only do we all need minerals in the proper balance, we also need vitamins. Imbalances in both vitamins and minerals can cause disease, pure and simple. Getting too much of a single vitamin or mineral can be just as dangerous as getting too little. Sometimes it's hard to know exactly what we need.

Here's the crux of The Vitamin Lie: Almost all vitamins sold on the market today are not vitamins. They are drugs. Yes, drugs! How could this be?

Let's start with a couple of simple definitions:

What is a vitamin? A vitamin is a naturally occurring essential nutrient that either the body manufactures or the body derives from food or other sources (such as sunlight in the case of vitamin D). Vitamins are complex molecules, combinations of enzymes, amino acids and various trace minerals.

What is a drug? It's a chemical compound that does not normally occur in the human body. Drugs are substances synthesized by laboratories. Drugs may have some basis in naturally occurring nutrients, but they have been synthetically or chemically altered, broken into pieces and are not biochemically identical to the naturally occurring complex vitamin molecules.

Vitamin C is a great example. Vitamin C is absolutely essential to human survival. We'll go into this in much greater detail in the coming pages, but vitamin C is not ascorbic acid, despite what most of us believe. Yes, ascorbic acid is one of many nutrients in the vitamin C molecule. Vitamin C molecules also contain P, K and J factors, tyrosinase enzyme, 14 known bioflavonoids, various ascorbigens, five copper ions, iron, manganese, zinc, selenium, phosphorus, magnesium, and yes, ascorbic acid.

That's just what we know about it. Nutrient vitamins like vitamin C are extremely complex molecules and there are probably dozens, if not hundreds, of other nutrients present in that molecule that we have not yet discovered.

The body is completely dependent on the whole vitamin C molecule. We cannot make it ourselves, so we must get it from our food in order for us to survive. There is no evidence that pieces of that molecule have any of the same effects as the whole C molecules. Ascorbic acid on its own may have some effects, like a drug. It has been shown to have some antibiotic-like effects, which would be good in some cases, but it also blocks the absorption of the whole C molecule, as well as interfering with its benefits and causing its excretion in the urine, depleting our body's stores of this important molecule.

But here's the economic reality: Almost all "vitamin C" on the market today is ascorbic acid or variations thereof. It says so right on the label in the parentheses, "Vitamin C (as ascorbic acid)." Why? Ascorbic acid is incredibly cheap to synthesize and/or isolate in a lab, with very little or no natural plant material.

Vitamins cannot be patented, so drug and supplement companies have no interest in producing quality, unpatentable, whole food products. They know we have bought into The Vitamin Lie and that most of us believe we must have "vitamin" C to prevent colds and a host of other maladies, so they know we'll buy it. What we don't know is that, at best, the ascorbic acid you bought at the drug store is doing nothing for you, and it is actually depleting your vitamin C levels. In some unique circumstances, it might even kill you.

"Vitamin" C is only one of the multitudes of so-called "vitamins" and their derivatives and combination formulas on the market today that qualify as drugs. They are not natural, no matter what the label says. These are only tiny pieces of the whole food that is the source of the vitamin you need. Vitamins are extremely complex molecules, most of them with more components than science has yet been able to detect. For example, vitamin A is actually a family of three groups of biochemical compounds (retinoids, retinols, and retinoic acids) and there are over 600 known forms of retinoids alone, with at least 19 of these found in the human body. Only one of these is the beta-carotene molecule, part of which is present in most synthetic forms of "vitamin A." These nutrient components work synergistically. In simple terms, this means that the whole is greater than the sum of the parts: Each little component of a vitamin molecule enhances the function of the others.

It's another "aha!" moment when we realize how whole foods are designed to contain all the nutrients our bodies need.

Think of it this way: If you take ascorbic acid or beta-carotene or another single component of a "vitamin," it's like taking calcium only when your body needs all 78 minerals for survival. Calcium is a necessary mineral for everyone, but to take calcium without all the other minerals or in excess is inviting disaster, as you've learned in the earlier chapters of this book.

Along the same lines, to take part of a vitamin without taking the whole vitamin invites similar disaster. Any vitamin you take should be carefully collected from whole foods that have been vine ripened in minerally balanced soil and picked at their nutritional peak. In addition, they should be alcohol extracted and processed without heat, which is a notorious destroyer of these delicate life-sustaining nutrients.

How do you know if your vitamins meet these requirements? That's the $64,000 question considering the artificial need that drug and supplement companies have created for products that aren't what they promise. Buyer beware! Your health is at stake.

Here are my suggestions:

- If the label doesn't tell you that your product is made from vine ripened, organically produced, alcohol extracted whole foods, without heat, it probably is not of the quality you are seeking. It is a drug.

- Here's a great clue: If the label says vitamin C (as ascorbic acid) or vitamin A (as beta carotene), don't waste your money. Those parentheses mean a substitution has been made; only one piece of the whole food is in your multi. If it costs $10 at your drug store, it definitely is not whole food or truly a vitamin and it may be harmful. Conversely, if it says 100% whole food and costs $30 to $70 at your local health food store, or enlightened doctor's office, it still may not be what you need, but you're on the right track. Whole food vitamins cost a bit more, but they are definitely worth it because you are worth it. To take anything else is to waste your money and possibly to jeopardize your health.

- Check out the resources section of this book and look at our website—www.calciumlie.com—for recommendations on quality products and for updates and expanded information.
- If you're in doubt and you have a product in mind, contact the company and ask about contents, growing conditions and processing.

Take your vitamins and minerals separately. Avoid multivitamins that have minerals added. They are usually undissolvable, poorly unabsorbed and they may be harmful to you, based on your tissue mineral levels. Your mineral needs should be determined by your hair tissue mineral analysis (HTMA). Your mineral intake should be carefully balanced so the vitamins can get the minerals where they are needed and both can do their jobs.

Don't pay attention to the government's RDAs or recommended daily allowances or RDIs, recommended daily intakes for "vitamins." I don't think anyone really knows the basis for these government-recommended amounts of "nutrients," but at least one author has theorized that they came from the nutrient profile of the needs of a World War I soldier, later revised and translated to women's needs without any scientific basis! How absurd! Considering the relative nutrient status of some 90-plus years ago, and the comparatively primitive nature of the laboratory equipment of the time, it makes absolutely no sense to make such a determination to apply to today's humans.

Today, the Food and Nutrition Board of the National Academy of Sciences meets every five years and sets or readjusts the RDAs. RDAs should not be confused with the needs or requirements for a specific individual. The key is to consume 100% whole food vitamins and balanced mineral supplements.

THE VALUE OF FOODS

Of course, you should eat foods that provide the greatest amounts of the nutrients you need, hopefully based on a reliable tissue mineral analysis. Vine ripened, fresh, fresh frozen, naturally dried and raw foods grown in minerally rich soils generally contain the perfect proportions and perfect balance of most of the nutrients we all need.

There are problems with this, as you might imagine. Few of us eat exactly as we should. Most of us eat what we like and do so repetitively. We eat what we grew up liking and what our parents fed us. We buy what we like every time we go to the store, so we grow up and develop "hereditary" nutritional medical problems. These are not inherited family medical problems, but a family-based nutritional shortfall translated into nutritional diseases.

It is difficult to avoid junk foods, fast foods and processed foods that are downright harmful to our health. Even if you're getting the greatest foods possible, grown locally without pesticides or other harmful chemicals, vine ripened and shipped a short distance to your table while the nutrients are still at peak value, you're still probably missing essential minerals and vitamins.

Having a well balanced diet with adequate minerals is a nice thought, but it's not very realistic. We already know that our minerally-depleted soil makes it nearly impossible to get all of our essential nutrients through food, and the majority of our food is not vine ripened. That makes supplements a necessary part of our nutritional system in order to make up the shortfalls. This doesn't mean you can compensate for a cheeseburger and chocolate cake diet by taking a few vitamins and minerals. Good nutrition is at the heart of good health.

So, OK, you've got your minerals balanced and now it's time to go on to the best vitamins. Here are the ABC's, and beyond, of what's good—and what's not.

ABC'S OF VITAMINS

There are five different classes of vitamin compounds or vitamin complexes. It's important that you remember that vitamins are complex and they are never, ever made up of one single nutrient.

Here are the A, B, C, D, E and F's of vitamins:

Vitamin A

Here's what vitamin A does:

- Maintains health of immune system;
- Regulates inflammation, tissue repair and wound healing;
- Formation of skin cells and mucous membranes throughout the respiratory, digestive, urinary and genital tracts;
- Formation of bones and soft tissues, including muscles, cartilage and ligaments;

- Assists in adrenal and thyroid gland function;
- Essential for good eyesight, night vision and corneal health;
- Formation of tooth enamel;
- Assists in maintaining a normal pregnancy and embryonic development;
- Assists in reproduction, fertility, lactation, sperm and egg formation;
- Supports nervous system;
- Protects liver.

Dietary sources of the fat soluble vitamin A include meat and cheese, red, orange and yellow fruits and vegetables, and dark green, leafy vegetables. Fish oils, egg yolk and butter are excellent natural fatty sources of this fat soluble vitamin.

Vitamin A is actually a complex family of nutrients that includes retinols, retinoic acid, and retinoids. There are actually over 600 known different kinds of retinoids, generally referred to as pro-vitamins, 19 different ones have been found in humans, among them a group called beta carotenoids.

Vitamin A is not beta-carotene, although that is what you'll see on most vitamin bottles: "vitamin A (as beta carotene)." Beta carotene is a drug and has, in fact, been shown to cause birth defects. The medical establishment has largely removed beta-carotene from prenatal vitamins because of its direct link to birth defects. This should have been a clue that something was wrong. Unfortunately, physicians have bought into The Vitamin Lie for so long, they didn't recognize the warning sign or the difference either. This shocked me when I first learned it since I too had been giving my patients prenatal vitamins with beta carotene in them without questioning the label.

This is another occasion for my "whole food" speech. It may be that the vitamin companies don't realize the fraud they are perpetrating on the American public. I'd like to think that is true, but I fear they are very aware that the products most of them are selling are ineffective or even harmful. They are drugs.

Too much beta carotene can cause birth defects, hair loss, cirrhosis of the liver, water retention, skin diseases and more unpleasant problems. Yet, you could drink carrot juice all day long, to the point where your skin turns orange, and while you might look a little strange, you wouldn't have any physical problems or cause your developing child to get birth defects. That's because the carrot juice is a whole food. The beta carotene found in carrots is a pro-vitamin or precursor of active vitamin A and is stored up in the body (liver, fat, and skin) and only converted to vitamin A as it is needed. Vitamin A has no known toxicity. It is 100% whole food and not a drug. This is one of the strongest examples we have in the difference of these chemically isolated compounds (drugs) and organic 100% whole food vitamins.

Vitamin B

Most of us know that vitamin B isn't just one vitamin, but most of us think there are just 12 B vitamins. You'd probably be surprised to know there are at least 56 vitamins in the B family. These water-soluble vitamins are known as B_1 (thiamine), B_2 (riboflavin), B_3 (niacinamide), B_5 (pantothenic acid), B_6 (pyridoxine). B_7 (biotin), B_9 (folic acid) and B_{12} (cobalamin). These vitamins are frequently referred to as B-complex, although most of the drugs sold as "vitamins" contain only these most common B "vitamins" and not the whole B vitamin complex molecules. While all of the components of the B-complexes can be separated, they always occur together in nature and no single B vitamin is ever found alone in a food.

Here's what the B-vitamins do:

- They have a vital function in cellular metabolism as co-enzymes to speed up biochemical processes;
- They help form DNA, the genetic material from which all cells are created and reproduce;
- They are necessary for the health and normal function of the nervous system;
- They maintain healthy skin, heart, liver, eyes, hair, spleen, thymus, pancreas, kidneys, red blood cell production and muscles;
- They stimulate digestion, secretion of digestive enzymes and insulin;
- They are essential for immune system function, resistance to infection and injury;
- They are a key part of endocrine gland system function (thyroid, adrenals, pituitary, ovaries and testes);
- Promote cell growth and division, including healthy red blood cells;

- They facilitate carbohydrate, protein and fat metabolism and cellular energy production;
- As a complex, they work synergistically to reduce and prevent stress, depression and cardiovascular disease.

B vitamins are found in clams, salmon, halibut, trout, salmon, beef, dairy products, brown rice, eggs, raw seeds and nuts, peas, avocados, nutritional yeast, bananas, oranges, grapes, pears, barley, oats, yams, corn, rye, dried beans, peppers of all types, dark green leafy vegetables, potatoes and tomatoes.

Strict vegetarians need B_{12} supplements, since the essential factor, methyltetrahydrocyanocobalamin, is found only in animal products.

Any kind of refining, cooking or processing damages the molecular structures of the B complex vitamins, which is again why raw foods are the best sources of vitamins.

I prefer to use raw seeds and nuts (use raw nuts only if you are at your ideal body weight because of their high caloric values), which contain good amounts of the B-complex vitamins undamaged by a heating process. Sprouts are also a good source of B-complex vitamins.

Would you pay for a tune up for your car and change only one spark plug? If you have several kids, would you feed only one? Would you pay for cable TV if there were only one channel? Taking only one B-vitamin is neither logical nor efficient. So avoid doing it unless there is a good reason. Get your B-vitamins from whole foods. There is such a close relationship between the various B-vitamins that a shortfall or excess of any one of this complex will affect the functions of all the other B-vitamins. Large doses of one of the synthetic "vitamins" can also create an imbalance and cause a relative deficiency of other members of the B-complex.

The need for whole foods is underscored by the story of World War II American troops held in Japanese prisoner-of-war camps who were being fed a diet of white rice only. They were getting beri-beri, a thiamine deficiency disease that results in nerve and heart damage, lack of coordination, numbness, stumbling gait, degeneration of nerve tissue, loss of reflexes, memory loss, loss of muscle tone, nausea, emotional instability, confusion, depression and leg edema. The situation became so dire that the Red Cross was given permission to bring in vitamin B_1 (thiamine) to help them. But the Red Cross vitamins didn't work, precisely because they contained thiamine alone. What did work? Tiny handfuls of rice bran given to prisoners by their more compassionate guards. The POWs found that four men could share one tiny rice bran kernel and get enough of the B-complex vitamins they needed to regain their health, at least enough to reverse the severe thiamine deficiency.

I think this example can be translated to many Westerners today who subsist on a diet of processed and nutritionally void foods with few nutrients, including B-complex. That gives us another explanation for the widespread depression, anxiety, fatigue, Type 2 hypothyroidism, intestinal disorders and adrenal insufficiency we see on our society.

The above is a brief discussion of only one form of B-complex vitamin. There are more than 50 B vitamins. It's important to understand that no natural vitamin exists as a single chemical entity. Separated from their whole food complex molecules, the single-structure chemical "vitamin" has had numerous co-enzyme factors removed that are essential for the actions of these vitamins in humans.

Vitamin C

We've already gone into vitamin C as an example, but this important nutrient complex bears further examination. Ascorbic acid, a component of vitamin C, serves as the molecule's antioxidant envelope, where it protects the other nutrients in the molecule from deterioration. Ascorbic acid is only as much representative of vitamin C as is the wrapper is part of your candy bar. It's holding in and protecting the "good stuff" inside.

Here's what the components of the vitamin C-complex molecule do:

- Rutin (also called the "P" factor) strengthens blood vessels and other collagen containing tissues, like cartilage;
- The "K" factor supports proper blood clotting, limits bruising and contributes to bone strength;
- The "J" factor supports the oxygen-carrying capacity of the blood to the benefit of all organs and tissues;
- Tyrosinase activates organic copper, allowing copper to function in stimulating metabolism, energy production, hemoglobin formation, thyroid hormone production and cholesterol metabolism;
- That copper also helps iron to be incorporated into hemoglobin for healthy red blood cells with the help of tyrosinase;

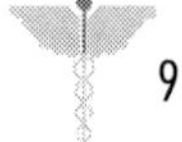

- The entire complex is key to all metabolic processes;
- It is involved in the formation of collagen, which forms connective tissues, gives them strength and is responsible for many cellular functions, including skin health and wound healing;
- Immune system function is dependent on vitamin C-complex;
- Hormone actions are dependent on C-complex;
- Assists in amino acid metabolism and absorption;
- Regenerates the active form of vitamin E-complex.

Vitamin C is found primarily in vine-ripened citrus fruits, berries, peppers, cantaloupe, broccoli, sweet potatoes, cauliflower, pineapple and mangos. Vitamin C is easily destroyed by heat, so it's best to eat these foods raw. All store-bought juices, whether fresh or frozen, have to be pasteurized by law. They are heated to 162° F for at least 30 seconds. This heat literally explodes the C molecule, completely destroying its nutritional value.

Vitamin C deficiency is probably one of the most significant health problems we face in our society today, largely because we've fallen prey to a subset of The Vitamin Lie, The Ascorbic Acid Lie. Our belief that vitamin C is ascorbic acid has led to an overall consciousness of some of the function of the C-complex molecule, including its role in immune function and healing. So, we pop a handful of ascorbic acid tablets at the first signs of a cold and think that will take care of the problem.

It was Linus Pauling, the brilliant Nobel Prize laureate, who woke us up to the value of vitamin C, but Pauling used whole vitamin C in his research, not ascorbic acid.

When you take ascorbic acid to ward off a cold, you are actually getting an antibiotic or drug-like effect of the drug ascorbic acid, not Vitamin C. You also deplete the whole food molecule, the real vitamin C-complex molecule, from your body, shunting it off along with all of its other beneficial parts in to your urine, without leaving behind anything good.

Conventional doctors pooh-pooh the idea that vitamin C deficiency is widespread in today's society. They think they haven't seen a case of scurvy in over 200 years since the link between citrus fruits and the sailors' vitamin deficiency was established and the potato blight of the 1800's occurred.

So what are the symptoms of scurvy? Thin skin, frequent bruising, bleeding from old wounds or even scars, purple swollen gums, bleeding gums, pale skin, fatigue, thinning hair, premature graying, poor wound healing and muscle aches and pains, among others. Doctors see it every day; they just don't recognize it.

Have you ever seen an elderly person with thinning hair and thin skin that bruises and breaks and bleeds easily? Perhaps she's losing her teeth or he's getting frequent nosebleeds. Of course, they'll complain of fatigue and body aches and pains. We're all related to someone like that and maybe we've even suffered some of those symptoms ourselves. Patients often tell me, "I bruise easily." All of these problems are signs of vitamin C complex deficiency and all of them are easily and quickly corrected with whole food C-complex.

You don't have to be elderly to experience C-complex deficiency. Vitamin C is crucial to the production of soft tissues, like cartilage and ligaments and tendons. We're seeing injuries to these tissues in many teenagers and people in their 20s and 30s. Joint replacement has become common in people in their 40s and 50s because of their weak and deteriorating soft tissues due to vitamin C deficiency. Back problems and herniated discs are the product of the same deficiencies.

In addition to your whole foods C-complex, you'll need to increase your intake of C-rich foods. I eat at least half an orange every single day, even though I know it came from Florida or California all the way to Alaska. Sorry, we just can't grow oranges in Alaska. The thick skin of oranges helps preserve the vitamin content and most oranges are tree-ripened before they are picked, since they won't ripen off the tree. I fortify my orange drink in the morning with fresh frozen rose hips I pick every year in Alaska, and fresh frozen raspberries also picked from my raspberry patch, along with rice bran and fiber added. It's so good!

I'll tell you a little personal story: Four years ago, I fell during a "home improvement" project. I completely burst or exploded the bone of one vertebra T9, and had a compression fracture of T12 and broke all the ribs in between. Doctors told me the chances were a million-to-one that I would ever walk again. I refused to accept that diagnosis because I knew some things they didn't. I had great faith and had been taking whole food C-complex for nearly four years by then. My disc tissue was so strong that it did not rupture. Even thought the bones were broken and literally exploded, the discs remained intact. My recovery was painful and slow, but I am fully functional, pain free and walking perfectly today. Walking is a blessing we so easily take for granted. In fact, I passed my military physical fitness tests, part of my Army Reserve officer's status while on active duty in Operation Enduring Freedom, less than two years after the accident. I continue to thank my God, my loving wife, many prayers and whole food Vitamin C-complex for my recovery.

Vitamin D

This oil-soluble vitamin is also a complex with at least 10 compounds in the D family, so it is important to get all the elements of vitamin D, not just one. Vitamin D-complex is essential to proper mineral metabolism. If you remember the composition of bones and the mineral storehouse function of bones from chapters 2 and 3, it's important to add here that vitamin D helps in the movement of minerals in and out of the bones as they are needed elsewhere in the body.

What else vitamin D does:

- Monitors excretion of calcium through the urine and maintains proper blood calcium levels;
- Helps minerals harden bones;
- Helps maintain bone growth;
- Helps keep the nervous system healthy by regulating calcium levels in blood;
- Plays a role in production and release of insulin to balance blood sugars;
- Works with parathyroid hormones to keep calcium at proper levels;
- Regulates cell growth and so may be protective against certain types of cancer, and may help prevent heart disease;
- Enhances immune function;
- Has a role in mood and depression;
- Contributes to muscle strength.

Vitamin D is a strange nutrient in that we get most of our supplies from sunshine on bare skin. This isn't very practical in January in Alaska, where I live, or even if you live in New York, Illinois or Minnesota. Heck, Kathleen says it's a bad idea in the mountains of North Carolina where she lives. Fatty fish (think salmon and tuna) are the main food sources of vitamin D, with cod liver oil as the huge winner on the vitamin D scale with an impressive 1360 IU per tablespoon.

We know that the body's ability to absorb vitamin D falls off as we age, and that the deficiency can result in osteoporosis. Studies estimate that 30 to 40% of elderly people with hip fractures are D deficient. Excess synthetic "vitamin" D, however, like the drug added to milk, can lead to excess calcium with the cascade of effects we already know about.

There is a Vitamin D Lie, too, unfortunately, that comes from the notion that synthetic vitamin D added to foods will make up for a shortfall. Synthetic vitamin D is like all the other so-called vitamins that are made from one element of a complex molecule. There has been a great deal of research on vitamin D recently and it is very promising, but we still don't know enough to take the risk of swallowing handfuls of supplements. In particular, synthetic vitamin D added to homogenized cow's milk has been shown to cause adverse effects on heart, muscle and artery cell walls, probably because of the excess calcium. Worse yet, one study showed that infant formulas fortified with synthetic vitamin D had excessive amounts of this drug/imitation vitamin.

The issue is how to get a dosage that will be sufficient without overdosing. Before deciding to take a vitamin D supplement, you need to know your calcium to magnesium ratios from a hair tissue mineral analysis (HTMA) and your overall tissue calcium levels. If you have an imbalance in your calcium/magnesium ratio, or a significant calcium excess in your tissues, Vitamin D and cod liver oil may be harmful to you, until you correct the imbalance. Taking this vitamin without knowing your levels, or taking it in large amounts, could greatly accelerate all the disease changes discussed in this book due to excess calcium. Your needs are also dependent upon your body fat levels because fatty tissues store up vitamin D. You should not take large amounts of vitamin D unless you know you need it by laboratory testing and you are paying careful attention to your relative intracellular calcium levels. The implications of vitamin D deficiency however are too significant to ignore this problem, even in the presence of a relative intracellular calcium excess. Although, replacement should be very judicious until the intracellular calcium levels are corrected.

This one is really a no-brainer. You can get what you need from sunlight, free of charge. It doesn't take a lot and you don't have to worry about skin cancer. Just go out in the sun with your face, head and arms uncovered, for less than ten minutes a couple of times a week and you'll be covered (pun intended). While our bodies can't store vitamin D for a very long period of time, this kind of exposure as often as you can do it will get you through most winters in the lower 48. In Alaska, we've learned the value of fatty fish, halibut, and salmon to help us get the vitamin D we need to get through those long winters.

Vitamin E

Vitamin E is the subject of yet another of these endless lies. The Vitamin E Lie goes like this: We need the alpha tocopherols in vitamin E as an antioxidant protection against a variety of diseases of aging, including heart disease, cancer and diabetes. The Vitamin E Lie is similar to the Vitamin C Lie in the sense that, much as ascorbic acid is only one part of the vast C-complex, alpha tocopherol is only one of a large number of complex compounds that make up vitamin E.

Vitamin E:

- Is essential to reproductive health. Lab animals deprived of vitamin E were infertile;
- Required for normal sexual development in both sexes;
- Is essential to the central nervous system, mental alertness;
- Part of the endocrine gland system and has a role in thyroid, adrenal and pituitary glandular function;
- Assists in controlling inflammation and repairing tissue damage;
- Participates in the maintenance of smooth, skeletal and heart muscles;
- Is involved in iron absorption and the production of red blood cells;
- Contributes to skin and hair health;
- Contributes to kidney, liver and lung health;
- Has a role in blood sugar metabolism;
- Has powerful antioxidant and free radical taming properties;
- And much more.

Vitamin E is found in raw nuts, raw seeds, unrefined cold pressed vegetable and nut oils, wheat germ, flax seed meal, green leafy vegetables, broccoli, liver, alfalfa and corn.

So, back to the Vitamin E Lie: Like all vitamins, vitamin E is a complex molecule with many components. The main components are tocopherols and tocotrienols, but among these two main categories, there are eight known forms of tocopherols and four known forms of tocotrienols, four essential fatty acids, selenium, lipositols and xanthenes. This is the same story as with other vitamins: Making a pronouncement that just one piece of such a complex vitamin is the vitamin is plain and simple dishonesty and can be dangerous to your health. This is also why many of the research studies on "vitamin E" have shown no effect or benefit, because researchers are using an inert drug, not the real vitamin E-complex molecule.

For some inexplicable reason, the original study on the "vitamin" E isolate was a rat fertility study using alpha tocopherol succinate. This study became the gold standard to determine how much of this substance was necessary to reverse infertility in rats fed a rancid diet. The naturally occurring vitamin E complex is a relatively stable molecule. The alpha tocopherol has been shown to have the strongest antioxidant property of all the tocopherols in the vitamin E molecule. In order to market the alpha tocopherol as "vitamin" E, the supplement companies must use a stabilization process called "esterfication," which gives the product a long shelf life and prevents it from becoming rancid or oxidized. This process makes the alpha tocopherol ineffective as an antioxidant in humans since it has been processed, so it won't interact with oxygen. It is biochemically inert or inactive in humans. It works in rats, however, because they have different biological processes. Therefore, alpha tocopherol has no antioxidant or vitamin E effects in this form in humans.

What's more, in one study, vitamin E deficient laboratory animals fed mixed tocopherols only died sooner than control animals who received no vitamin at all.

Another study, this one on humans, showed that a low concentration of vitamin E in the blood plasma was a greater risk factor for death from heart disease than was elevated cholesterol or high blood pressure. This should have been a clue, that scientists were testing a drug, not a vitamin. Yet, we need vitamin E to survive. What's the answer?

This one is simple, and cheap, too: Get your vitamin E from raw nuts and seeds, from unrefined cold pressed vegetable oils or 100% whole food vitamin E supplements.

Vitamin F—essential fatty acids

OK. There is no such thing as vitamin F, although it is a name once attached to the need for the healthy fats we all need. Anyway, it fits neatly into our alphabet soup of vitamins and it makes them easier to remember. We all need vitamin F (essential fatty acids) and, sadly, it is another part of The Vitamin Lie. We all need unsaturated fatty acids, sometimes called UFAs, or unsaturated fatty acids.

Yet, sometime in the early 1980's, we as a nation got into a fat phobia. I'm not sure who started the idea that all fats are bad and that all fats make you fat. Nothing could be farther from the truth. However, we all started eating low-fat everything. Not coincidentally, we then started gaining weight. If you look at the graphs of the national obesity epidemic, its beginnings can be traced to exactly this same time period. We decided that it was OK to eat ice cream by the gallon, as long as it was low fat. Nothing slowed our national craving for French fries and our intake of lethal trans fatty acids went through the roof. We got supersized, literally. We now face dealing with a new "generation XL."

We all need fat in our diets. Without it, we die. Every one of the trillions of cell membranes in our bodies has two layers of fat and only one layer of protein.

The key is we need the right fats, the UFAs that come from unrefined cold-pressed vegetable oils, raw nuts and seeds rich in linoleic and linolenic acids and the Omega-3s that come primarily from deep water fatty fish and flaxseed.

Here's what UFAs do for you:

- Protect our hearts by controlling cholesterol and triglyceride (blood fat) levels and minimizing disease-causing inflammation;
- Combine with cholesterol and protein to form the membranes that hold cells together;
- Help transport oxygen to all cells and tissues;
- Establish normal growth patterns in children;
- Improve mental and neurological health by easing depression and anxiety and enhancing attention and learning abilities;
- Keep brain cell communication healthy, reducing the risk of Alzheimer's disease;

- Slow the course of arthritis and ease chronic pain and inflammation;
- Improve the course of pregnancy, promote healthy outcomes for the mother and long term physical and mental health for her child;
- Promote healthy physical and mental development for our children;
- Enhance energy production;
- Produce hormones;
- Lubricate skin, our largest organ.

The earliest sign of fatty deficiency is often dry, red, itchy skin and the onset of dermatitis and other skin diseases.

We get our vegetable-sourced UFAs from raw nuts and raw seeds and oils made from them. Most UFAs are destroyed by any heat over 160 degrees Fahrenheit, so roasted nuts and seeds and heat-processed oils are nutritionally without value and potentially toxic. Check your labels carefully, because most oils are processed with heat and chemical solvents. The label should say your oil is cold pressed, unrefined or expeller processed, not cold processed, which includes heat in the process as well as cooling.

We get Omega-3s primarily from fatty fish like salmon, tuna and cod. Omega-3 is also present to a somewhat less usable degree in flaxseed, some cold pressed vegetable oils and green leafy, vegetables.

The Omega-3s in fish oil are the most common source of these essential fats and two major elements are responsible for the health benefits:

- **DHA** (docosahexaenoic acid) has many positive effects, but perhaps the most impressive is its ability to help lower triglycerides. High triglycerides are linked to heart disease in most, but not all, research. Research also shows that DHA is important for helping pregnant women carry their babies to full term and gives their babies the maximum nourishment through breast milk, for visual and neurological development in infants, learning in young children, normalizing brain function, emotional and psychological well-being, preserving eyesight, insulin resistance (pre-diabetes and diabetes) and easing digestive and reproductive difficulties.
- **EPA** (eicosapentanoic acid) is credited with reducing excessive blood clotting that can lead to heart disease. EPA also plays a role in reducing stress, keeping physical energy levels up, eye health and good brain function.

Alpha linoleic acid, a third element of the Omega-3s from plant sources, is converted to DHA and EPA in the human body, but the transition is inefficient, so it requires approximately ten times the vegetable-sourced Omega-3s to receive the amount of DHA and EPA found in salmon, tuna or other coldwater fish, best eaten as unheated or raw sushi to get the maximum nutritional value.

Most fish oil products on the market are genuinely made from fish oil, so the composition of the product is not in question; it is the source and the processing that can be problematic. Mercury and heavy metal contamination are serious concerns for anyone who eats fish caught almost anywhere in the world. Wild-caught Alaska salmon is one of the few exceptions to this rule. Farmed fish are not worth your money because they are fed an unnatural diet that limits their Omega-3 content and the farming methods include toxic chemicals that contaminate the fish as well as the ocean and even wild fish in the vicinity. There are supplements that are processed in such a way that they are safe and any heavy metal contamination is removed. Among them is a shark liver oil product I like with amazing healing properties, but there are probably others as well. Molecularly distilled products also have a high degree of purity.

FINALLY . . .

I wish I could say to you, "Take this multi or this individual vitamin or that mineral formula." I can't. There are some very good products on the market, and some are even excellent. But there are very few I can unequivocally recommend as the perfect product and none that can be considered the save-all and end-all of all products. I approach all supplements the same as I am trained to recommend medications. I want the best for my patients, the best for their needs and their budgets. But most importantly, I want what helps my patients get better. Whole food is a very important key, as is balance. Know your balance and imbalance, know your needs and excesses and eat as if your life and health depends on it. It does. Take a look at the resource section of this book and check in with us regularly at our website, www.calciumlie.com, as we add new product recommendations and updates to material in this book. We welcome reader recommendations through the website so we can expand our list of recommended products.

POINTS TO REMEMBER

- A vitamin is a naturally occurring essential nutrient that the body either manufactures or derives from fresh food or other whole food sources.
- A drug is a chemical compound that does not normally occur in the human body. Drugs are substances synthesized or isolated by laboratories. Drugs may have some basis in naturally occurring nutrients and may even be marketed as "natural," but they have been synthetically or chemically altered. They have effects, some good and some bad.
- Almost all "vitamin" supplements on the market today are actually drugs.
- All vitamins are complex molecules. Avoid any "supplements" that are made of only one ingredient, i.e. so-called vitamin C that is composed exclusively of "(ascorbic acid)." These are drugs, not vitamins, and they can be harmful or have drug-like effects.
- The multiple nutrient components that compose a vitamin molecule act synergistically, each enhancing the effects of the others.
- There are medical myths about what each of the most common vitamins should be. Despite the depletion of our soils, it is still possible to get most of our essential vitamins from food. Your vitamins and supplements should all be made from vine- or tree-ripened whole foods. End of story.

CHAPTER 8

The Road Back to Health

SO NOW YOU'RE ARMED WITH A LARGE VOLUME of information and perhaps more biochemistry than you'd like. We've made it as painless as possible and only burdened you with what you absolutely need to take action. When we're facing lies, information is our only weapon. You may have to read the earlier chapters more than once in order to assimilate the information we have presented here.

Now is the time for action.

This is your action plan to find your way back to health.

It won't happen instantly, although you'll probably notice some changes in a matter of days. Perhaps you'll feel more energy or some simple symptoms, like dry skin or restless sleep, will smooth themselves out. There will be bumps in the road, detours and days when you feel like all the effort isn't worth it. All we can say is, "Keep going." I remember a sign I once saw that said, "When you're going through hell, keep on going." You will come out the other side and be healthier and stronger for the experience. If there is a little discomfort along the way, it's a small price to pay for avoiding the major health problems that our society has come to associate with aging.

It's possible to be vibrant and healthy when you're 20, 30, 40, 50 or far beyond. It is possible to be 60 or 70, 80 or even 90 and free from heart disease, diabetes, dementia, cancer, cataracts and canes. It is never too late to start. I have 60-, 70- and even 80-year old patients beginning this program and loving it.

At the beginning, your road back to health will take some extra focus, but it will become second nature within weeks. Take it a day at a time and do what you can.

Little changes make big differences. You had to learn to crawl before you could stand, stand before you could walk and walk before you could run. You probably fell down a few thousand times at first. To keep doing the same thing and expecting different results is insanity. Improve one thing and you will improve two, two and you will improve four. Getting more healthy becomes a congruent lifestyle.

If you only follow the program and improve one meal a day, you'll be 33% successful. That's highly significant in scientific terms. If you do what I am asking for two meals a day, that is 66% success. That's off the charts in terms of scientist's gauge of results and you will get those kinds of changes if you stay with the program. If you adopt this plan as your lifestyle and adhere to it 99% of the time, your results will be beyond your imagination. I'm living proof of this. I'll tell you more about that in Chapter 9.

FOOD IS STILL THE FOUNDATION

The great news: A very significant part of your road back to health will come from eating the right foods. You can get a large percentage of your necessary nutrients—vitamins and minerals—from food. Choose the right foods, according to your tissue mineral analysis food recommendations and your return to health will be far less expensive in economic terms than if you rely entirely on supplements.

This may seem like a contradiction of our earlier statements, but despite the depletion of our soils, food is still the best source of unrefined carbohydrates, protein, vitamins (when they are made from vine-ripened foods), minerals and most of the nutrients we need. Humans cannot live on supplements alone, no matter how high the quality!

Based on our current food growing and marketing practices, I believe supplements are essential and we especially need minerals.

As much as possible, eat vine-ripened organic foods. You'll still have to add supplements, but this will give you the best possible sources of vitamins and minerals from your food.

Here are a few great ways to get your vitamins through whole food:

- Eat an orange a day for whole food vitamin C, or blend it with fiber, rice bran and fresh frozen raspberries (my favorite) or fresh frozen rose hips (these are very plentiful in Alaska).

- Enjoy $\frac{1}{4}$ to $\frac{1}{2}$ cup of raw pumpkin and sunflower seeds for essential fats, vitamin E and B vitamins. Mix your seeds with organic raisins or cran-raisins for vitamin C and potassium.
- Eat as many vegetables as possible every day (not including potatoes) and vary the types of fruits and vegetables you eat. Minimize the amounts of fruit you eat and maximize your vegetables.
- Use unrefined, unprocessed sea salt or rock salt liberally. Remember, this type of salt contains all minerals in perfect proportions. Table salt is essentially zero nutrition.

While this type of diet may not give you every single nutrient you need, it will go a long way toward promoting the best health you can achieve.

Go organic as much as your budget will allow. Buy locally produced foods when they are available because their nutrient content will be higher. Don't let the lack of a budget for organic foods or locally available produce be a stumbling block for you. Do what you can. Anything you do will help your body.

Start to think of food as the best possible nourishment for your body. Anything you put in your body should be dedicated to your return to health.

Fresh foods are almost always best, although there is some argument in favor of frozen foods, which are picked at the peak of their ripeness and quickly preserved by freezing. Avoid canned foods except tomatoes and beans. The high heat in the canning process destroys nearly all vitamins and minerals in foods and the cans can be the sources of toxic minerals like tin and aluminum. Tomatoes and beans are an exception to this rule. Certain vitamins and fiber are actually released during the cooking and canning processes for these foods.

Avoid pasteurized foods as well, since the heating process of pasteurization destroys enzymes, vitamins and nutrients.

Most foods are best eaten raw or cooked very lightly. Steam or lightly sauté, bake or broil foods.

Avoid the microwave like the plague! Microwaves destroy most of the nutrient value in foods and make them worthless. Portuguese researchers found that broccoli zapped in the microwave with a little water lost 97% of its antioxidants, while lightly steamed broccoli only lost 11%.

Best, yet, eat the major proportion of your fruits, vegetables, nuts and seeds raw.

I love the idea of pulverizing raw vegetables in a high speed blender. This soup (never heated above 120 degrees Fahrenheit, or better yet, not heated at all) offers our bodies the most absorbable nutrients possible. Add a little organic chicken broth, a clove or two of garlic, a dash of cayenne and it's a delicious quick meal in a glass.

I don't recommend juicers. They take out the fiber, a very important part of our diet. Always eat fruit 30 minutes before or two hours after protein and never eat it with a regular meal.

Shop often and buy small amounts so you'll have the freshest possible foods on hand. The longer a food remains in the refrigerator, the more nutrients it loses.

If you have the space and the inclination, grow some of your own food. Every little bit helps. You have complete control over the garden and you can keep toxic chemicals out, even if you have to sacrifice a small percentage to the birds and the bees and other critters. Even a tomato plant on an urban balcony or a jar of alfalfa sprouts on a New York apartment window can serve as an inspiration to keep your feet on the road to health. There are few greater pleasures on this Earth than biting into a sun-warmed tomato you just harvested from the garden you planted with your own hands.

Take some time to savor and appreciate your food. There was actually a study of prisoners fed a really terrible diet of prison food. Those who gave thanks for their food, in whatever spiritual tradition they preferred, actually gained more nourishment from that food and had far fewer physical illnesses than those who simply chowed down.

And speaking of chowing down, do take time with your meals and chew your food thoroughly. Chewing and mixing our food with the digestive enzymes in saliva while it is still in your mouth is the first part of the digestive process. If you are swallowing large chunks of barely chewed food, you'll gain little nourishment from it. Think of your mouth as that high speed blender and pulverize your food into small pieces so you can get the maximum nutritional value from it.

Also, as a general rule, don't drink with your meals, drink before or two hours after. This extra fluid dilutes your digestive enzymes and decreases your digestion of your food.

GETTING STARTED

You'll need a hair tissue mineral analysis. This is really the only way you can determine your exact mineral status and from that, learn what you need to do to improve your health.

I've said before, the only laboratory that I recommend for an accurate HTMA is Dr. David Watts' Trace Elements Inc. in Addison, Texas. This lab adheres to the highest possible standards and I absolutely trust their results.

Dr. Watts is a brilliant scientist whose database of 800,000 HTMAs shows distinct patterns for various deficiencies and toxic ratios of key minerals. This extensive data pool gives scientific validation to the links between mineral deficiencies and imbalances and manifestations of disease, ranging from high blood pressure to osteoporosis to thyroid dysfunction, and more.

You need to get an HTMA from Trace Elements Inc. through a HTMA health care provider who uses this lab, since Trace Elements, Inc. will only accept samples submitted by physicians. The report will be much more meaningful with help from a trained health care professional to guide you to the correct ways to address imbalances.

Correct collection of the hair for the HTMA is a must. Please carefully follow the collection directions.

We are gathering a list of practitioners who regularly send samples to Trace Elements for HTMAs and this will be included on our website, www.calciumlie.com. Be sure to check back often, since the list will certainly expand and other resources will change as we find more resources to help you.

SIX STEPS ON THE ROAD BACK

Here are six steps I consider most essential for good nutrition. Do these and you'll be well on the road to great health and long life.

1. Drink pure water

Water is the stuff of life. Most of us need more than we drink. Everyone needs at least 64 ounces of water a day, more if you are overweight, a heavy exerciser or live in a very warm climate. As a general rule, we need to drink one half of our body weight in ounces of water. For example, if you weigh 150 pounds you would need to drink 75 ounces of water daily, or two and one half quarts of pure water every day. Remember 72% of your body's weight is water and you need to keep that balance in order to be healthy. Water helps sweep toxins from your body.

Get the purest water you can. If you have municipal drinking water, consider buying a good quality filter. These can cost anywhere from $200 for a quality counter top filter to $3,000 for a whole house filter. As a general rule, filters that have a carbon block filter that is changeable put glue in the water because the carbon is glued to hold it into the filter. I recommend pressed carbon block without glue. I think the best product is manufactured by Sun Aqua Systems. See www.calciumlie.com for ordering information.

This topic is hugely complicated. Take your time and identify your specific water needs carefully. Your life depends on it.

Avoid bottled water since much of it is little more than tap water put in a plastic bottle that will expose you to xenoestrogens that leach from the plastics. Plastic bottles are also environmentally unfriendly and extremely overpriced. For the same reason, drink all of your water from glass containers. If that is impossible when you are traveling, buy a stainless steel water bottle and carry filtered water from home or take a filter with you on your trip.

Never drink distilled water, which has had virtually all contaminants, nutrients and the very life of it removed. To do so also increases your mineral requirements.

And think of the water you bathe in. Your skin is the body's largest organ and it absorbs toxins or nutrients. If you are showering in chlorinated water, the warm water opens your pores and your body literally drinks in the chlorine and other contaminants and brings them into your body. Ditto for hot tubs. If a whole house water filter isn't in your budget, you can buy an inexpensive shower filter that will cost you less than $10 a month.

2. Take ionic sea salt derived minerals

In nearly 1,000 patients I have tested in my practice, there has been only one person who had a near perfect mineral balance. (It wasn't me!)

We all need minerals and virtually none of us get enough. Ionic minerals are the only ones that are completely available for our bodies to use because they are water soluble and they naturally carry an electrical charge that allows them to be carried through the cell membranes.

Besides the trillions of functions they perform in our bodies, these minerals are the transport system for vitamins and amino acids, so without them and without minerals in balance, these nutrients can't get into our cells and our bodies simply won't function as they should.

See the resource section for my recommendations on ionic mineral supplements. Sadly, there aren't very many I can recommend in good conscience. I'm always looking for more quality recommendations, so if you know of high quality ionic sea-salt-derived mineral products or 100% whole food vitamins, please contact me via the website, www.calciumlie.com.

The best source of ionic minerals is in unrefined sea salt and rock salt, if you do not already have a sodium excess on your hair tissue mineral analysis. Sodium excess in an HTMA is typically a stress pattern or a false elevation related to water softeners. This is the case in fewer than 10% of all tissue mineral analysis results in my experience. Add harvested pure sea salt liberally to your foods and forget the myth about salt causing high blood pressure. That's nonsense! High blood pressure is caused by excess calcium and amino acid deficiencies, as we discussed at length in Chapters 2, 3, and 4.

3. Whole food vitamins

Almost all of us need supplements because we simply aren't getting our full complement of vitamins and minerals from our food.

Many of us need additional supplements to help correct imbalances and deficiencies and to treat specific disease conditions.

Avoid vitamins made from anything but 100% whole foods that have been vine ripened. All store-bought "vitamins" are drugs and, unless you have a specific purpose for taking them in drug form, they will not help you, and they can potentially harm you. I use them in specific circumstances to achieve balance according to the HTMA results and specific recommendations from the Trace Elements lab.

As we have discussed throughout this book, essential whole food vitamins are the only way to ensure you will get all of the complex molecular elements of these nutrients. You need all of the nutrient components together in their whole food form to get the full benefits. Some vitamins have dozens, and possibly even hundreds, of specific nutritional components. We may not even know about some of them yet, as more and more are being discovered every year. We do know that many of these elements work synergistically, meaning that they enhance one another's effectiveness. That is the best argument I can think of for 100% whole food vitamins that contain all the components with which foods were designed.

We have the same problem recommending whole food vitamins since there are so few on the market. Check the resource section of this book and check in frequently on our website, www.calciumlie.com, since we'll be adding new information as I hear about new products that I can recommend. I currently recommend Innate pure vitamins, as these are the only ones I can confirm are 100% whole food.

The best natural sources of readily available vitamins include raw seeds. Raw seeds have all known B complex vitamins (remember there are more than 50 of them), E complex, and essential fatty acids. Also eat dried, frozen or vine-ripened fresh fruit for vitamin C-complex in its whole food form. Almost all store-bought fruits and vegetables are not vine ripened and, therefore, have little mineral content and virtually no vitamins. The correct form of supplements can reap huge benefits.

4. Essential fatty acids

The correct form of essential fat is vital to human health. Every cell membrane in our body has two layers of fat and only one layer of protein. When The Fat Lie made us paranoid that fat would make us fat, we derailed our nutrition and actually triggered weight gain. The historic obesity charts released by the Centers for Disease Control and Prevention substantiate that the beginning of the low fat diet craze in the early 1980s corresponds exactly to the upward trend in obesity in the United States.

Get your essential fats from the best possible sources. There are two essential fatty acids that we need: Omega-3 in the form of alpha linoleic acid, or ALA, and Omega-6 in the form of alpha-linolenic acid, or GLA. These two are considered essential because humans can't manufacture them within our bodies.

Eat raw nuts and/or seeds daily. They are excellent sources of essential fats—the good kind that you need every day. In 2003, the FDA approved the following health claim for seven kinds of nuts:

> "Scientific evidence suggests but does not prove that eating 1.5 oz per day of most raw nuts as part of a diet low in saturated fat and cholesterol may reduce the risk of heart disease."

However, if those nuts are roasted, they lose almost all their nutritional value and become toxic. Always opt for raw nuts (and seeds, for that matter). In any case, limit your intake to not more than 2 ounces daily. (We know it's hard to stop once you start popping those delicious raw cashews or almonds.) However, if you are above your ideal body weight, opt for raw seeds only, and skip the nuts.

- Raw pumpkin seeds are particularly good sources of essential fats as well as zinc, iron, calcium and phosphorus, with some magnesium and copper. There is a mix of complex vitamin E and B vitamins, with niacin being the richest in pumpkin seeds. Sunflower seeds are also very high in potassium, low in sodium, with healthy levels of zinc, iron, calcium, copper, manganese and phosphorus. They also have substantial levels of the essential amino acid methionine which helps to detoxify the body, activate enzymes and improve cellular energy production.
- Raw sunflower seeds are rich in B complex vitamins and one of the few naturally occurring food sources of vitamin D. Always opt for raw seeds and limit your intake to ¼ cup daily. Those individuals with a high tissue copper level should temporarily avoid these and opt for pumpkin seeds instead.
- Use cold pressed oils made from nuts and seeds (extra virgin olive oil and cold-pressed sesame oil are particularly good). Heat processing destroys the delicate structures of the fat molecules, rendering them virtually void of nutrition. After heating, the fats become rancid and toxic. We all know what that would do to our cars; our bodies are the most important cars we drive. Treat them well. Put the best possible oils in them. The best oils are expeller pressed. Avoid "cold processed" oils. This is a marketing gimmick and deceptive. It means they were cooled somewhere along the process. Good cold-pressed oils will indicate on their packaging that they have been processed without any heat or chemicals.
- Get healthy fats from wild fresh caught cold water fatty fish like salmon, halibut and tuna. Eat them at least once a week, twice a week is better if you're sure they come from a mercury-free source. If you're not sure, ask.

There is no equal to fresh Alaska wild salmon or halibut. Sushi is truly the best way to receive these omega-3 fatty acids which cooking essentially destroys. Raw fish needs to handled very carefully to avoid bacterial contamination.

5. Eat high quality proteins

The protein we humans get in our diets primarily come from meats, seafood, eggs, beans, chicken, game meat, duck and turkey. These protein sources are the source of the essential amino acids that are the building blocks of every protein molecule, hormone, neurotransmitter, cell membrane middle layer and immune molecules and important to the biologic function of every cell in the human body.

We must get these amino acids from proteins we eat every day, since we cannot store them for later use.

A shortfall of just one of the 10 essential amino acids can result in deterioration of the proteins inside the body. Your body will actually "rob" amino acids from muscle tissue to make up for a shortfall.

There are at least 10 essential amino acids that are necessary for critical bodily functions and at least a dozen or more additional amino acids that play hugely important roles in human nutrition and metabolism.

Essential amino acids are phenylalanine, valine, arginine, threonine, tryptophan, isoleucine, methionine, histidine, leucine and lysine. The other most important amino acids are cysteine, glycine, glutamine and tyrosine.

Our primary sources of amino acids are meats, seafood and eggs, which contain all of the amino acids necessary for our survival. Eggs, in fact, contain the protein source most similar to human protein.

Incomplete proteins can be obtained from sprouted grains, raw nuts and raw seeds. Vegetarians, particularly vegans who do not eat any animal protein, must pay close attention to combining protein sources so that the full complement of amino acids is part of their diet every day. For example, a homemade raw peanut butter sandwich on a sprouted grain bread such as Ezekiel bread, black beans and brown rice or a bean burrito made with a sprouted grain tortilla would make a complete protein meal with all the essential amino acids. Unfortunately, vegans commonly suffer from severe mineral deficiencies and generally lose digestive enzyme capabilities over time.

Choose your meats, seafood and eggs carefully. When at all possible, buy organic meats and poultry that have been produced without antibiotics or added hormones or chose game meat.

Be careful not to mix fruit and protein in the same meal, which causes the protein to ferment in the gastrointestinal tract, releasing alcohol into the blood stream causing yeast overgrowth in the intestines and, in some cases, in the blood stream. This is considered a bad food combination. Fruit should be consumed one half hour before protein or two hours after eating protein.

Buy wild caught seafood from cold waters where heavy metal pollution is diminished. Seafood is a good source of protein and essential fats.

For most of my patients, I recommend avoiding or minimizing dairy products, since dairy products are high in calcium, and since most of us have calcium excess, we don't need these calcium-rich foods. Also remember, eggs contain only HDL (the good cholesterol) and no bad (LDL) cholesterol. This is the third most common nutritional lie. Be careful to cook your eggs without oil of any kind and you will get 100% good fat. Our brains are about 70% good cholesterol. Don't eat egg substitutes; there is no good reason for this. It is how you cook your eggs and what you eat with them that is the problem. For example, it is the bacon, sausage, cheese, or eggs fried in margarine, olive oil or butter that gives us the bad LDL fat.

6. Get essential monosaccharides

This is probably a new recommendation for most of you and it's a subject of our next book, so bear with us while we enter some uncharted territory. Every protein molecule in the human body is dependent on monosaccharides for its action(s). Monosaccharides, the simplest form of carbohydrate molecules found in the body, are absorbed through the intestinal wall and carried in the bloodstream to tissues where they may be stored or used, in some cases, as an energy source.

On the biologically active end of every protein molecule is a complex monosaccharide receptor. These receptors are quite literally the keys that unlock every biochemical reaction in the human body, ranging from the formation of DNA and RNA to blood type, the creation and action of insulin, the action of all hormones, and every cell membrane receptor. Without the monosaccharide keys and the correctly fitting monosaccharide locks, things just don't work.

Monosaccharide deficiencies are implicated in nearly all abnormal autoimmune responses whereby immune molecules, called immunoglobulins, become abnormal immunoglobulins. This takes place when there is a nutritional deficiency of monosaccharides. These immune molecules literally pile up because they can't find a receptor to bind to. Eventually, they become foreign proteins triggering an autoimmune reaction in the body. This process then causes the immune system to attack these molecules and/or normal healthy tissues. Monosaccharide deficiencies have been shown to be a factor in several autoimmune diseases such as systemic lupus erythematosis, rheumatoid arthritis, juvenile rheumatoid arthritis, ankylosing spondylitis, scleroderma and Sjogren's syndrome.

In one study, patients with autoimmune diseases were compared to matched controls of patients without the diseases. Each of the autoimmune diseases studied was found to have specific deletions and/or substitutions of at least one specific monosaccharide on a specific immunoglobulin protein molecule receptor that was exactly the same in all affected patients, with a huge statistical significance. The medical profession has largely ignored this data because it didn't make sense or lead to a drug therapy. After all, their way of thinking is if you have one of these illnesses, you couldn't have a nutritionally-derived illness, so you must have a steroid drug deficiency. This is, of course, completely illogical.

It seems hard to believe that one simple sugar molecule could make that much difference or create that much havoc in the human body.

However, the entire difference between blood types A, B, AB and O is only one simple monosaccharide molecule on the terminal receptor that specifies your blood type. We have long ago recognized what happens if you receive a transfusion of the wrong blood type, especially a second time. It will potentially kill you. This creates a whole new perspective about the significance of monosaccharide deficiency.

These monosaccharide deficiencies are preventable. A teaspoon of maple syrup every day in your oatmeal or fruit smoothie is a good way to add monosaccharides.

Between the ages of 20 and 60, our bodies lose 70% of our receptor protein activity, due to the depletion of the number of monosaccharide receptors on the ends of each and every protein molecule in our bodies. This causes our biochemical reactions to run less efficiently. It is like changing from a jumbo jet to a two-cycle gas engine. Both engines work, but one is 70% efficient, the other is around 30% efficient. Which would you rather have flying your airplane?

When we're young, we have sufficient enzymes and cofactors to complete the nearly 16 steps it takes to convert the more complex sugars into the various other monosaccharides, such as fucose. As we age, this process becomes less efficient and is no longer driven to completion. Healing becomes slower, hormones less efficient and, in some cases, immune diseases such as cancer and autoimmune diseases such as lupus and diabetes, develop because our immune responses and cell membranes lack the correct receptors.

Monosaccharides are divided into four major types of sugars: glucose, glucosamine, galactose and galactosamine and four lesser known sugars: fucose, xylose, acarbose and manose. For the most part, they do not occur in our diets. For our purposes in this book, there are very few good natural food sources of monosaccharides, but you will find them in some fruits, berries, melon, some root vegetables like sweet potatoes, parsnips, beets and onions, in honey and pure maple syrup and other tree sap syrups. I believe tree sap syrup (pure organic maple syrup) is the best source for the money.

You don't need to eat large amounts of these foods to get the monosaccharides you need. A handful of strawberries, half a small sweet potato, a fresh onion on your burger or a teaspoon of maple syrup in your morning oatmeal should do the job quite nicely for most people under the age of 40.

It's also available in a supplement form and, if you're over age 40, I think it's a good idea to include this in your supplement regimen. If you're over age 60, or if you have any type of autoimmune disease, you need to add monosaccharides.

A multilevel company, Manatech, also markets monosaccharides in a powder form called Ambrotose. I believe that their product is overpriced and they have been guilty of falsely advertising their content of monosaccharides, however, they do have a good source of at least 6 essential monosaccharides. Another company, Improve U.S.A., Inc., marketing pure stabilized aloe vera-derived product, may be a good alternative. See our resource section and visit our website, www.calciumlie.com for updates and further information.

HOW MUCH WILL IT COST?

We'll be the first to admit, the cost of supplements and better quality foods can be pricey. You know your budget, but please do think of this program as an investment in a longer, healthier life. Prioritize your budget with this in mind.

With some employers, you can set up a medical savings account that will allow you to pay for supplements in pre-tax dollars. That'll save you anywhere from 15% to 35% right off the top, depending on your tax bracket. You can also pay for your HTMA and consultation with your doctor from these funds without having to hassle with your insurance company.

Some insurance companies will pay for these tests and almost all of them will pay for a nutritional consultation. It's certainly worth filing a claim. In my experience, no other test has the potential to change your health more significantly.

When it comes to supplements, don't waste your money on so-called "supplements" that are actually drugs unless there is a specific need or indication. There may be times that those supplements are appropriate in a short-term situation, but like any prescription drug, their use should be as minimal as possible and for the shortest time possible. Use only whole food products and go for the best. It will pay off in the long run in terms of your health and your pocketbook, too. See the Resources section or refer to our website, www.calciumlie.com, for my recommendations.

Budget and prioritize what you need to make a difference in your health. I find so many patients are already spending money on supplements that are not helping, I feel that it is part of my job as a physician to direct my patients to what is good, what will make a difference and what works.

Finally, we urge you to do what you can. Start with baby steps and you'll soon find yourself walking and finally, running.

We admit, the HTMA results and nutritional recommendations that accompany them can be a little overwhelming. Don't let yourself be overwhelmed, but take the advice of the old saws: How do you eat an elephant? Answer: One bite at a time. Little changes in food buying preferences based on HTMA results and thoughtful supplementation can bring about amazing results.

Take charge of your health and take control of your life. Do what is important and do it well. You can make a difference in your health and regain vitality and energy in ways you never imagined were possible.

One additional note: I find that there is nothing better than walking 30 minutes a day to decrease stress, improve circulation and build relationships. This is truly remarkable! You will become closer to the person you walk with in every case. Exercise is almost always good, but walking has many more benefits than almost any other form of physical activity.

POINTS TO REMEMBER

- Little changes based on HTMA results can produce big results over time. Improving one meal per day is a 33% improvement, two meals 66% and three meals, 99% improvement.
- Remember the six essentials to good nutrition. If any one of these is missing from your diet, there will be consequences, some immediate and some later: pure water, adequate minerals, essential vitamins in the whole food form, essential fatty acids, protein or essential amino acids and essential monosaccharides.
- The HTMA from Trace Elements Inc. will have an incredible impact on your health. No other medical test has a greater chance to impact your health long term. No other company has the correct levels and ratios to make this test absolutely meaningful and reliable. It is never too late to get started. Go to www.calciumlie.com for more information.
- Budget for supplements and take the ones that are the most important and most likely to have the greatest impact on your health. They are, unfortunately, necessary today due to the nutritional deficiencies of our foods.
- Walking is great for decreasing stress and building relationships.

CHAPTER 9

Doctor to Doctor: An Impassioned Plea

THROUGHOUT THIS BOOK, WE'VE THROWN OUT some—ahem—unconventional ideas about health, nutrition and the underlying causes of the diseases that are quite literally shortening our lives.

Everything in this book is based on solid, scientific evidence. There's nothing airy-fairy or mystical about it. Most of the premises in this book come from basic biochemistry, courses every doctor took in pre-med and medical school.

We'll be the first to tell you that these concepts are not well known or commonly accepted. Patients who take them to their doctors are likely to be summarily dismissed or even ridiculed. Doctors who espouse these common sense, solid scientific concepts are likely to be ostracized by their colleagues. I know. I was a victim of that sort of professional jealousy and jousting.

Patients, by all means read this chapter and read it closely. But we have really written this concluding chapter as an open letter to all doctors, an impassioned plea for them to put aside their prejudices and their adherence to The Calcium Lie, The Vitamin Lie and a dozen other erroneous belief systems that are not scientifically based.

We urge you, with our blessings, to copy these pages of this book and give them to your doctor. Make your pleas for your physician to read these pages as impassioned as is our advocacy for you.

We know doctors are busy people, so we are making this chapter short and sweet to economize on valuable time, but doctors, we urge you to buy a copy of this book and read it in its entirety. We think it will change your life, your practice and be of great service to your patients. Who knows? Maybe it'll even help you improve your health and heal yourself. The basic truths in this book are irrefutable.

A LETTER TO ALL DOCTORS

The majority of physicians practicing today are there because they made a choice to help people. I felt the same way. I was a bright-eyed, naïve, idealistic youngster who, at age 19 felt a special calling to the practice of medicine. Almost all of us had those altruistic motives when we entered medical school, but the way medicine is practiced today, those altruistic motives have been largely beaten out of us.

I know, I've been there. It's a lot like being a hamster on a wheel. You have to keep turning that wheel to stay ahead. Despite what most laypeople believe, a license to practice medicine is not a license to print money. In fact, there is absolutely no security in practicing medicine. It is basically a service occupation with high overhead and high risk of legal liability and very little security. Maybe I should call this The Big Bucks Doctor Lie.

Sure, some doctors are earning beaucoup bucks, but the average doctor is confronted with huge debts, big overheard expenses, enormous insurance premiums, no paid time off to rest, vacation and recuperate and no retirement benefits.

And we are expected to be knowledgeable about everything medical, make snap decisions when we are exhausted and always be right. Yes, you can make a comfortable living, but you have to work hard for it and make sacrifices that most people would never consider.

If you're on that hamster wheel and feeling overwhelmed, go back to those days when you were a bright-eyed med student. It was your choice to become a physician. In my 31 years of practice, I've discovered something that borders on the mystical: Enough money keeps on coming as long as I work hard and make the right choices, even in the hard times, and yes, I have had them too. As long as I keep my sights on my mission to help my patients feel better and get better, all is well.

I have been the victim of professional jealousy, anti-competitive behavior, vicious gossip and professional attacks by colleagues who felt threatened by my success. The behavior I have witnessed and experienced firsthand is despicable, to say the least.

In 1996, I was ready to throw in the towel, stop competing with my colleagues, give up on the insurance companies and quit medicine for good. I had no idea what I would do, but I was just sick of the way many in my chosen profession cannibalize each other over money, with totally uncompassionate and anti-competitive behavior, in the name of good medicine. Sometimes, unfortunately, a physician or group of politically entrenched physicians protect and cover up substandard practice behaviors arbitrarily and capriciously, in the name of peer review and and financial gain.

It was on one of my lowest days as a physician that a phone call came informing me that I had been chosen one of the "Best Doctors in America". What an honor! My spirits soared in a conflict of irony and my thoughts of leaving the profession were diminished. Maybe I could make a difference. Maybe I could take whatever criticism and heat my colleagues could dish out as long as someone recognized that I was actually doing what was right, what I had originally set out to do. I was helping my patients get better and it was being recognized nationally. Amazing.

At about the same time, I realized that I had been developing an increased awareness and intellectual accountability for my pregnant patients who would come in and ask me about the nutritional supplements they were taking. They wanted to use various herbs and supplements, as well as pre-natal "vitamins" and they wanted my recommendations about the best ones to take and how much was safe.

These are the same questions we face as physicians every day concerning drugs. I realized that I needed to practice the same due diligence by educating myself about nutritional concepts and supplements that weren't even in the books when I was in med school or, at least, not in the ones we studied. I also needed to go back to my roots in basic science and biochemistry and apply what I did know to human nutrition and separate fact from fiction.

I'm pretty sure your experience in med school was similar to mine: We got four hours or less of instruction on human nutrition out of thousands of class hours. Doctors are not "supposed" to have to know this stuff. Yet this information is quite literally at the heart of how we treat our patients, no matter what our specialties. Virtually every disease process of the human body has a connection to nutritional imbalances, toxicities, shortfalls and deficiencies. Yet we spend so little time learning about nutrition that we have to re-educate ourselves.

I was not only re-energized in my practice of medicine, I felt compelled to research other fields of medicine and nutritional products so I could provide my patients with the best possible care and guide them in what was safe, what works, what doesn't and what not to take. I started to learn more about herbs, supplements and other alternative therapies, including homeopathy.

Before you pooh-pooh homeopathy, think about it. The use of homeopathy or microscopic doses of various toxins or non-toxic substances to trigger an immune or physiological response works because these remedies are water soluble and can be carried into the cells easily. Think about your basic biochemistry and homeopathy will make sense to you. More importantly, it has been used for over two hundred years, has a scientific basis and, when used properly, it does no harm. If it works, great, use it. If it doesn't work some of the time, try something else. There is ample evidence-based medicine that it works. In my experience, homeopathic remedies work about 80% of the time to treat symptoms. Remember, drugs don't always work either.

I discovered that there was an amazing amount of medical knowledge regarding the use of herbs in medicine which are often the basis for our drugs. They have various effects, good and bad, some even stimulate immune responses, but like homeopathy and drugs, herbs largely treat symptoms but with less toxicity.

That was when I discovered The Calcium Lie and its links to mineral deficiencies and excesses. In a nutshell, The Calcium Lie says that bones are not made of calcium, but of at least 12 minerals, including calcium. Expecting to keep bones strong by giving someone calcium supplements is like expecting that you can make a loaf of bread from yeast alone. It simply won't work and, in the case of calcium supplements, it can do great harm as crystallized excess calcium concretions make their way into arteries and joints and force the adrenals to compensate for calcium excess to their own detriment.

We're not going to re-hash this entire book here, but we're going to repeat The Calcium Cascade from chapter 2 here, since you may have received these copied pages from a patient (with our blessings) and you may not yet have access to the entire book. The chart may help trigger some recollections for you of how the biochemical process we describe in this book is perfectly logical, based on the biochemistry classes you took in medical school.

It leads to a simple conclusion: Almost everyone needs trace minerals, not just calcium, because we simply cannot get all nutrients we need through food grown in minerally depleted soils, picked before ripeness, especially in view of our society's propensity for nutritionally void foods. And most importantly: calcium hardens concrete, not bones. Excess calcium can do severe damage to the human organism.

When I resurrected my old biochemistry textbooks, I discovered The Calcium Cascade. It triggered insatiable curiosity in me. I began to quickly build my knowledge about nutritional supplements, something I am somewhat ashamed to confess I had pooh-poohed to my patients before then. I discovered what worked and what didn't. I had to struggle to overcome the brainwashing I had received on The Calcium Lie. I dug deeper and I found out about hair tissue mineral analysis, how reliable testing methods could provide me with a wealth of information about a patient's medical conditions and how to address them nutritionally.

I began to look at the cost effectiveness of the treatments. If one treatment wasn't working, I searched for alternatives and networked with other like-minded professionals to find out if they had any answers. I continue to do so.

I also became acutely aware that I was being forced to label patients with their afflictions. Someone with diabetes became a diabetic and was labeled accordingly. That's how we are trained. But as I began to change my way of thinking, I realized that there are no diseases we are "supposed" to have and that almost all of these labels are related to nutritional deficiencies and imbalances which, when corrected, cause the illnesses to remit. It opened a whole new way of thinking for me, a whole new approach to my patients, and helped them immeasurably. That's so much more like what I'd originally set out to do.

As a little aside, I'll tell you that as soon as I began to change my way of thinking about diabetes and started treating the nutritional and mineral deficiencies and imbalances in patients with Type 2 diabetes and insulin resistance, I began to achieve phenomenal success.

Over the past 12 years, my treatment plan has kept blood sugars normal in more than 80 patients with diagnosed Type 2 diabetes over long periods of

The Calcium Cascade

Excess calcium in the human body begins a cascade of negative effects that have enormous adverse consequences to our health. This process cannot be diagnosed with standard blood tests. It requires a reliable, competent lab to conduct a tissue mineral analysis on a correctly collected hair sample you provide. I recommend Trace Elements Inc., the only lab with the correct ratios and databases. You can find information about them in the resources section and through my website, www.calciumlie.com.

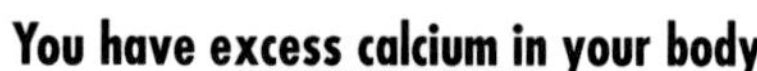

You have excess calcium in your body

THAT LEADS TO

Calcium seeking more magnesium to try to keep your body in balance

THAT LEADS TO

A relative magnesium deficiency in proportion to calcium that leads to increased muscle tension, and nerve endings firing erratically and other "electrical" functions of the body malfunctioning;

AND

In its need for more magnesium, your body has to suppress adrenal function in order to retain more magnesium to compensate for the high calcium, causing a loss of sodium and potassium in your urine;

THAT LEADS TO

A continual depletion of the sodium and potassium that are stored inside the trillions of cells in your body;

THAT LEADS TO

A loss of the sodium and chloride you need to produce the stomach acid you need to digest protein;

AND

This increases the incidences of heartburn and other digestive disorders, and the use of prescription drugs that have further destructive effects and impede digestion;

AND

Your body gradually loses its ability to digest protein and absorb the essential amino acids that are the building blocks of protein.

ALSO

the sodium depletion leads to failure of the sodium pump, the mechanism by which our bodies get essential amino acids and glucose into our cells, not including fat cells;

FURTHERMORE,

Potassium levels decline dramatically—this leads to thyroid hormone resistance and slowed metabolism;

SO

All cells (except fat cells) become starved for glucose

RESULTING IN

increased cravings for glucose and for minerals leading to more cravings

AND

deficiencies of sodium, potassium, and essential amino acids, and more cravings.

THE END RESULT IS:

Multiple metabolic malfunctions, including, obesity, heart disease, Type 2 hypothyroidism, Type 2 diabetes, anxiety, migraines, depression, hypertension,

and the list goes on and on!

time. It is effective for virtually everyone with insulin resistance if caught and treated early on in the course of the disease. Based on my experience, if the diagnosis has taken place in the past two years, Type 2 diabetes is always reversible. If the diagnosis is five years old or less, Type 2 diabetes is still sometimes reversible. If the diagnosis has been made more than five years in the past, my treatment plan may not be able to reverse the disease, but it can result in improved blood sugar control.

Joe R was one of these patients with recent onset Type 2 diabetes. His fasting blood sugars were from 150 to 250 and post prandial sugars from 250 to 350. With immediate and correct supplementation, within two weeks, all his blood sugars were normal and have remained so for more than 12 years.

For Joe and these other patients, the key was correct supplementation with the appropriate supplements to reduce insulin resistance, not just sensitizing the body to the overproduction of insulin, which increases fat cell glucose absorption. That means treating and reversing the underlying problem with the correct supplements, not drugs. Chromium picolinate doesn't work (see Chapter 5), but chromium polynicotinate (ChromeMate™) does.

I don't expect the dairy and pharmaceutical industries and the supplement companies will like this book much, since it is challenging you to think and move away from the erroneous belief systems they have so carefully nurtured. No doubt, I will be attacked for my unconventional ideas. It's OK. I have pretty broad shoulders and thick skin.

We have struggled in the writing of this book to put these concepts into simple terms that the average reader can comprehend. If we have oversimplified, we will take responsibility for that. Of course, biochemistry is very complex. There is no doubt that physicians are among the most intelligent people in the world, and we know you can take these simplified concepts and apply what you learned in medical school to acknowledge their truth.

I take intellectual honesty with great seriousness. I cannot have a knee jerk reaction to a patient's question about a supplement, medication, surgery or any type of treatment. That knee jerk reaction would be based on what I think I know and not necessarily on science. I continually take myself back to my roots in med school biochemistry and ferret out the answers based on science, not advertising or drug rep dinners or just "knowing" something.

Before this goes too far, I want to say I don't consider supplements to be a panacea. In fact, many supplements are actually drugs, and as such can be harmful. This is the subject of Chapter 7 of this book, The Vitamin Lie. The

Vitamin Lie says that we've been duped into believing that a single component of an extraordinarily complex molecule that comprises a vitamin is the vitamin itself. Case in point: Vitamin C is not ascorbic acid, although most vitamin C supplements sold on the market today are just that. Unless someone takes in the whole vitamin C molecule made from 100% whole foods, vine ripened and grown in minerally rich soils, your patients won't be getting the benefits of this remarkable vitamin.

This is my plea to you: Remember your roots. Remember who you are and how you were trained. Remember your early education, especially your biochemistry, however painful this may be.

Put aside belief systems about medicine and open your mind to what some may think are "new" ways of thinking, but which are actually just basic, solid science.

I remember a fairly pompous med school professor who told us that only 20% of everything that we were going to be taught was true. The only problem was that he didn't know which 20% was true—and neither did we. Maybe that one caveat contained more wisdom than I realized at the time.

Erase The Calcium Lie from your mind. You know that bones are not made of calcium and osteoporosis is the loss of minerals from the bones, not just the loss of calcium. Then treat your patients accordingly. See that they get a complete complement of trace minerals based on basic scientific evidence, and based further on hair tissue mineral analysis from a reputable laboratory. After all, isn't bone mineral density just another way of measuring tissue mineral levels, in this case, in bone? Think about it.

The only lab I trust completely to accurately measure whole body tissue mineral levels is Trace Elements, Inc. (www.traceelements.com or by phone at 800-824-2314 or through my web site at www.calciumlie.com).

Dr. David Watts, founder of Trace Elements, Inc., has developed a database of more than 800,000 hair tissue samples from which he has extrapolated highly accurate predictions of disease risk based upon the basic science of relationships of mineral deficiencies, excesses, imbalances and toxic ratios to known clinical disease and medical science. Find out your patients' mineral deficiencies and imbalances and you'll be able to begin treating them nutritionally with reliable, reproducible and gratifying success.

When you re-arrange your thinking process, you can treat your patients as you did when you were a bright-eyed med student. Begin to question what you think you know.

You can re-energize your practice of medicine, care a little more about your patients and actually help them get better, rather than just treating their symptoms as the pharmaceutical industry would encourage you to do.

Not everything that comes from the drug companies is good—nor is it all bad. We need to educate ourselves to discern what is good and what is not. No one else will do it honestly and it is our sworn responsibility as physicians.

We as physicians have great power to help or to hurt. It is our choice how we will treat our patients and how we will, ultimately, make a difference in their lives, our lives and the world. If you use this information with honesty, honor and integrity, you'll attract more patients than you can imagine. My ob-gyn practice has morphed into a practice that is about 50% nutritionally based, with many men and children joining my women patients.

This book is a gift to you. Take and use this information with our blessings for you and your patients.

Resources

Since we're forging new territory here, the resources we can offer are not as complete as we would like them to be. We hope that in the coming months and years, we'll be able to flesh out this list and offer you more resources for everything you need to combat The Calcium Lie and find your way back to health.

The best way for you to keep up with the latest information is to visit www.calciumlie.com often and subscribe to our newsletter at www.calcium lie.com/newsletter.

I know there are many other good products on the market. I have included in this list the products that I know and trust through my years of clinical practice.

Websites: www.calciumlie.com
www.aurorahealthandnutrition.com
Phone toll free: 877-260-6914
www.drt-obgyn.com

WHERE TO FIND A GOOD DOCTOR

- First, check our website, www.calciumlie.com. We hope to post an ever-growing list of physicians who are equipped to help you.
- The American College for Advancement in Medicine, an association of integrative health practitioners: www.acam.org, phone: 949-309-3520.
- The American Academy of Anti-Aging Medicine (A4M), which has doctors worldwide who are dedicated to preventive health: www.worldhealth.net, phone: 773-528-1000.

- Insulin Potentiation Therapy website: While this website is dedicated to a specific form of alternative cancer treatment, the medical doctors who administer this treatment are open-minded and likely to be able to help you to re-balance your minerals: www.iptforcancer.com

HAIR TISSUE MINERAL ANALYSIS (HTMA) TESTS

This test is the starting point of your journey back to health. It helps you determine your exact mineral status. While there are other labs that provide this test, Trace Elements Inc. is reliable, trustworthy and accurate. I use no other lab for this test. You can order the test through my website and get a consultation to help you understand the results and apply the recommendations that accompany your test results.

Learn more at: www.calciumlie.com
www.aurorahealthandnutrition.com

NATURAL SEA SALT

These are the best brands of natural and unrefined sea salt:
Celtic sea salt: www.celticseasalt.com
Redmond sea salt: www.realsalt.com (available in supermarkets and health food stores and through www.aurorahealthandnutrition.com)

VITA-MIX

A Vita-Mix machine is much more than a blender. It can process fruits, vegetables, even grains so that you can easily assimilate the maximum nutrients available in your food: www.vitamix.com

SUPPLEMENTS

www.aurorahealthandnutrition.com • Toll Free: 877-260-6914
www.calciumlie.com
www.drt-obgyn.com

The following list offers other companies and products I recommend. For specific information regarding their use in my practice, please refer to www.aurorahealthandnutrition.com.

Pro-Thera
Alpha Lipoic Acid: 100 mg tabs
Chromate 200 mcg tabs: 100 and 500 bottles
DHEA: 25 mg and 50 mg caps
Eciosamax ultra-pure omega 3 gel caps
Glucosamine: 750 mg capsules
5-HTTP: 50 mg caps
Indole Forte: 400 mg caps
MSM: 750 mg caps
Taurine: 500 mg
Thera PMS

Manatech (control #456515 to order)
Ambrotose Powder (plain)
Emprisone Cream

Innate
B-complex (100% whole food)
C-complex (100% whole food)
E-complex (100% whole food)
Pre/Post Natals (100% whole food)

Life Extensions
Cognitex

Research Nutritionals
CoQ_{10}
NT Factor Energy
Transfer Factor Multi Immune

Sanesco
Contegra
Lentra
Prolent
Somni TR

Corvalen
D-Ribose

Natural Partners
7 keto-DHEA: 25 mg and 50 mg
Eurocel
Germanium
Rhyzinate
Vitex

Wayne Garland
Diabetic Glucose Control Formula
Imperial Chi
Ocean Gold (shark liver oil)
Tolerance
Topical Shark Liver Oil

Klearsen Corporation
Eczema Relief Cream

Matol (control#21564298)
Fibersonic
Isogenix

Thorne Research
L-Tyrosine
Perfusia (sustained release L-arginine)
SF 722
SF 734

Body Health
Metal Free

Chi Enterprises
Myomin
N-HRT
Prostate Chi

Nurti Rice
Rice Bran

The Grain Society
Celtic Sea Salt

Probiotic
Thera Biotic Lactobacillus

Trace Mineral Research
Trace Minerals (blue-standard formula)
Electrolyte formula (red-extra potassium in standard formula)

TRACE MINERALS IONIC SEA SALT DERIVED MINERALS:

I like the ionic minerals produced by a company called Trace Minerals Research because I know they are safe, absorbable and effective. I admit they are a bit difficult to find, so I am offering them through my website. There are a couple of other products that are of good quality, so I'm including them here. You can also get them through my website.

www.aurorahealthandnutrition.com
www.mineralresourcesint.com
www.traceminerals.com
www.originalquinton.com

WHOLE FOOD VITAMIN C

Innate Vitamin C (100% Whole Food Vitamin C). This product is sold through doctors' offices. You can get it at my website.

www.aurorahealthand nutrition.com

WHOLE FOOD VITAMINS

I'm still searching for a 100% whole food vitamin that does not contain minerals. The Innate company is supposed to be developing one according to my specifications. Check my website and I'll post a specific product as soon as this one is available or I find another acceptable product.

www.aurorahealth andnutrition.com

MONOSACCHARIDES

Ambrotose—Manantech
Control number: #456515

www.aloewholesale.com (Improve U.S.A., Inc.)
www.aurorahealthandnutrition.com

This is the only monosaccharide product I have been able to find. If anyone knows of other products, please let us know through our website, www.calciumlie.com.

MAPLE SYRUP (FOOD SOURCE OF MONOSACCHARIDES)

Look for products that are 100% pure maple syrup, including:

www.dennisfarmsmaple.com
www.maplesource.com

TO TREAT SPECIFIC CONDITIONS

REFLUX AND GERD

Rhyzonate: www.aurorahealthandnutrition.com

HYPERTENSION

Profusia (sustained release L-arginine)
Ocean Gold (shark liver oil)

www.aurorahealthandnutrition.com

TYPE 2 DIABETES: CHROMEMATE™, DIABETIC GLUCOSE CONTROL FORMULA

www.aurorahealthndnutrition.com

ESSENTIAL FATTY ACID DEFICIENCIES

Eciosamax (ultrapure omega 3) (www.aurorahealthandnutrition.com)
Ocean Gold (shark liver oil) (www.aurorahealthandnutrition)

OTHER PRODUCTS

WATER FILTERS

Aquasana: www.aquasana.com
Jonathan Beauty Water Filtration: www.jonathanproduct.com/home.html
www.aurorahealthandnutrition.com

References

NOTE TO READERS

While there is good scientific research to back the theories presented in this book, all of the principles of The Calcium Lie, the effects of mineral deficiencies, insufficiencies and excesses are found in basic biochemistry. Any college biochemistry textbook will confirm every word in this book, extrapolated logically. This is why I am so dismayed that physicians who have studied these basic scientific truths in depths choose to "forget" what they learned in medical school and buy into these medical myths.

BOOKS

Anderson, F. *Nature's Answer—Replenish The Earth*, (Replenishing Press, Bear River, Utah, 84301, 2001).

DeCava, M. L. (1997). *The Real Truth About Vitamins and Antioxidants* (Brentwood Acadmeic Press, 1996).

Lee, John, *What Your Doctor May Not Tell You About Menopause* (Warner Books 1996).

Russell, M. R. *What the Bible Says About Healthy Living.* (Regal Books, 2001).

Starr, M. M., *Hypothyroidism, Type 2, The Epidemic.* (New Voice Publication, 2005).

Wallach, Joel and Lan, Ma, *Rare Earths, Forbidden Cures* (Wellness Publications, 1994).

Watts, David L. , *Trace Elements and Other Essential Nutrients.* (Writer's B-L-O-C-K, 2006).

Wright, Jonathan and Lenard, Lane, *Why Stomach Acid is Good for You* (M. Evans and Co., 2001).

Wright, Johnathan V. and Morgenthaler, John, *Natural Hormone Replacement* (Smart Publications, 1997).

(Dr. Wright has written several excellent books on natural healing.)

ARTICLES

CHAPTER 2

Statins

McLean, DS, Ravid, S. et al. Effect of statin dose on incidence of atrial fibrillation: data form the Pravastatin or Atorvastatin Evaluation and Infection Therapy-Thrombolysis in Miycardial Infarction 22 (PROVE IT-TIMI 22) and Aggrastat to Zocor (A to Z) trials. *American Heart Journal* 2008 Feb;155(2): 298–302.

Aspartame

http://www.mercola.com/article/aspartame/weight_gain_myth.htm

1. According to an article in Technology Review, "aspartame may actually stimulate appetite and bring on a craving for carbohydrates" (Farber 52).
2. An article in Utne Reader claims, "researchers believe that any kind of sweet taste signals body cells to store carbohydrates and fats, which in turn causes the body to crave more food" (Lamb 16).
3. From the San Francisco Chronicle, Jean Weininger states that "studies have shown that people who use artificial sweeteners don't necessarily reduce their consumption of sugar—or their total calorie intake. . . . Having a diet soda makes it okay to eat a double cheeseburger and a chocolate mousse pie" (1/ZZ1).
4. "The American Cancer Society (1986) documented the fact that persons using artificial sweeteners gain more weight than those who avoid them" (Roberts 150).

The major selling point of aspartame is as a diet aid, and it has been demonstrated that the use of this product actually causes people to consume more food. Normally, when a significant quantity of carbohydrates are consumed, serotonin levels rise in the brain. This is manifested as a relaxed feeling after a meal. When aspartame is ingested with carbohydrates, such as having a sandwich with a diet drink, aspartame causes the brain to cease production of serotonin, meaning that the feeling of having had enough never materializes. You then eat more foods, many containing aspartame, and the cycle continues. Monsanto's profit from its NutraSweet Division was $993 million in 1990.

Diet soft drinks, Type 2 diabetes

http://www.ajcn.org/cgi/content/abstract/82/3/675?maxtoshow=&HITS=10&hits=10&RESULTFORMAT=&author1=hu&searchid=1&FIRSTINDEX=0&sortspec=relevance&resourcetype=HWCIT

Aspartame insulin release

Liang Y, Maier V et al. The effect of artificial sweetener on insulin secretion. II. Stimulation of insulin release from isolated rat islets by Acesulfame K (in vitro experiments). Hormones and Metabolic Resistance 1987 Jul;19(7):285–9.

http://www.nih.gov/news/radio/aug2007/08102007soda.htm

Are you a middle-aged adult? Do you drink more than one soft-drink per day? It doesn't matter if it's diet or regular. According to a study by the National Heart, Lung and Blood Institute at the National Institutes of Health, you may have a more than 40 percent greater rate of either having or developing metabolic syndrome-that's a cluster of conditions that increase the risk for heart disease

Stellman SD and Garfinkel L. Patterns of artificial sweetener use and weight change in an American Cancer Society Prospective study. *Appetite* 1988;11 Suppl 1:85–91. (This is the seminal study in this field)

http://www.webmd.com/diet/news/20050613/drink-more-diet-soda-gain-more-weight

This scientific data was presented to the American Diabetes Association in 2005 by researchers from the University of Texas—lead researcher Sharon Fowler—but no paper has ever been published.

Fowler's team looked at seven to eight years of data on 1,550 Mexican-American and non-Hispanic white Americans ages 25 to 64. Of the 622 study participants who were of normal weight at the beginning of the study, about a third became overweight or obese.

For regular soft-drink drinkers, the risk of becoming overweight or obese was:

- 26% for up to ½ can each day
- 30.4% for ½ to one can each day
- 32.8% for 1 to 2 cans each day
- 47.2% for more than 2 cans each day.

For diet soft-drink drinkers, the risk of becoming overweight or obese was:

- 36.5% for up to ½ can each day
- 37.5% for ½ to one can each day
- 54.5% for 1 to 2 cans each day
- 57.1% for more than 2 cans each day.

For each can of diet soft drink consumed each day, a person's risk of obesity went up 41%.

CHAPTER 3

Bolland MJ, Barber PA et al. Vascular events in healthy older women receiving calcium supplementation: randomized controlled trial. *British Medical Journal* 2008 Feb. 2;336(7638):262-6.

Seely S. Is calcium excess in western diet a major cause of arterial disease? *International Journal of Cardiology* (1992 May;35(2):281-3.

Seely S. Possible connection between milk and coronary heart disease" the calcium hypothesis. *Medical Hypotheses* 2000 May;54(5):701-3.

Seely S. The connection between lactose and coronary artery disease. *International Journal of Cardiology* 1994 Oct;48(2):199-207.

Seely EW, Graves SW. Calcium homoestasis in normotensive and hypertensive pregnancy. *Comprehensive Therapy* 1993;19(3):124-8.

Seely S. Is calcium excess in western diet a major cause of arterial disease? *International Journal of Cardiology* 1991 Nov;33(2): 191-8.

Seely S. On arterial calcification. *International Journal of Cardiology* 1997 Sep 19; 61(2):105-8.

CHAPTER 4

Grinwald P. Sodium pump failure in hypoxia and reoxygenation. *Journal of Molecular and Cellular Cardiology* 1992 Dec;24(12):1393-8.

Seely S. The Connection between milk and mortality from coronary heart disease. *Journal of Epidemiology and Community Health* 2002 DFec;56(12);958.

CHAPTER 5

Dolidze NM, Kezeli DDF et al. Changes in intra- and extracellular Ca2+ concentration and prostaglandin E2 synthesis in osteoblasts of the femoral bone in experimental hyper- and hypothyroidism. *Bulletin of Experimental Biology and Medicine* 2007 Jul;144(1):17-20.

Grinwald P. Sodium pump failure in hypoxia and reoxygenation. *Journal of Molecular and Cellular Cardiology* 1992 Dec;24(12):1393-8.

Seely S. The Connection between milk and mortality from coronary heart disease. *Journal of Epidemiology and Community Health* 2002 DFec;56(12);958.

CHAPTER 6

Dolidze NM, Kezeli DDF et al. Changes in intra- and extracellular Ca2+ concentration and prostaglandin E2 synthesis in osteoblasts of the femoral bone in experimental hyper- and hypothyroidism. *Bulletin of Experimental Biology and Medicine* 2007 Jul;144(1):17-20.

CHAPTER 8

Bond A, Alavi A et al. The relationship between exposed galactose and N-acetylglucosamine residues on IgG in rheumatoid arthritis (RA), juvenile chronic arthritis (JCA) and Sjögren's syndrome (SS). *Clinical and Experimental Immunology* 1996 Jul;105(1):99-103.

Panzironi C, Silvestroni N et al. An increase in the carbohydrate moiety of alpha 2-macroglobulin is associated with systemic lupus erythematosus (SLE). *Biochemistry and Molecular Biology International* 1997 Dec;43(6):1305-22.

Bond A, Alavi A et al. A detailed lectin analysis of IgG glycosylation, demonstrating disease specific changes in terminal galactose and N-acetylglucosamine. *Journal of Autoimmunology* 1997 Feb;10(1);77-85.

Index

About the Authors

Dr. Robert Thompson is a board-certified obstetrician and gynecologist who practices in Soldotna and Anchorage, Alaska. While he is technically a "women's doctor," his work to expose The Calcium Lie has brought him many patients who fall outside his specialty. In fact, now more than half of his patients come to him for nutrition counseling and many of them have found long-term relief from chronic disease, including obesity, diabetes, hypothyroidism and adrenal fatigue. He happily counts among his patients many men and children as well as women who seek out his assistance as a gynecologist as well as a nutrition specialist.

He received his medical training at the University of Kentucky and has practiced in California, Pennsylvania, Hawaii and Alaska.

Dr. Thompson lives in Soldotna, Alaska, with his three labs, Ruger, Mystika and Zack, where he takes great delight in fly fishing, hunting, hiking, canoeing, water and snow skiing, snow machining, playing concert violin and raising and training Labrador retrievers.

Kathleen Barnes is a widely traveled journalist with more than 35 years of experience in publishing, print and broadcast media. In recent years she has specialized in medical, health and sustainable living for national magazines and newspapers and as author, co-author and editor of 13 books.

She has lived in Europe, Asia and Africa and brings a broad international perspective to her writing.

Kathleen lives in the mountains of western North Carolina with her husband, Joe, and two dogs, two cats and two horses.

CPSIA information can be obtained at www.ICGtesting.com
Printed in the USA
BVOW071238280512

291220BV00007BA/51/P

9 780981 581859